SICK

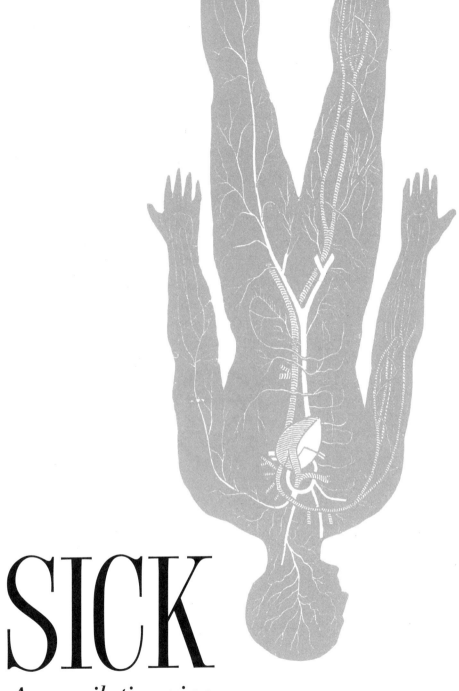

SICK

*A compilation zine
on physical illness*
edited by Ben Holtzman

Sick: A Compilation Zine on Physical Illness

Edited by Ben Holtzman
Designed by Carl Williamson

Distributed in the booktrade by AK Press
Available through Ingram and Baker & Taylor
at standard discounts

Microcosm Publishing
222 S Rogers St.
Bloomington, In 47404
812-323-7395
www.microcosmpublishing.com

We have other zines, books, patches,
stickers, buttons, shirts, and more at
www.microcosmpublishing.com

This is Microcosm #76099
ISBN 978-1-934620-48-9

Proofread by Sparky Taylor

INTRODUCTION

I was diagnosed with cancer in 2007 and had a recurrence in 2008. This zine developed out of a personal frustration during these times over the lack of discussion about and understanding of illness within radical/left/DIY communities as well as the lack of resources within these communities for those dealing with illness.

Too often those of us who are living with illness have felt that our experiences are not welcome in conversation, even within radical/alternative communities. Illness is considered taboo; it's seen by many as awkward, if not depressing, to bring up. This zine collects peoples' experiences with illness to help establish and further a personal and collective voice of those impacted by illness.

This collection is meant for several audiences. It is intended to be a document of experiences with illness that others in similar circumstances can relate to and hopefully take something from and thereby ease some of the isolating aspects of illness. It is also meant for those within our communities who have not directly experienced illness themselves. While no one piece – or even any one collection of pieces – can come close to encapsulating all experiences with and perspectives on living with illness, these writings are meant to increase understandings of illness and expand opportunities for dialogue.

While the types of illness discussed in this zine vary widely, it is striking how many of the pieces, in one way or another, mention support. Most commonly, this is in reference to *not* receiving adequate care and understanding from those around us. Illness is often misunderstood and, in some cases, ignored completely. In addition to the many pieces that bring up personal experiences with support, this zine also includes articles that focus on receiving support, providing support, and building supportive communities. While, again, the collective strength of these pieces does not wholly reflect the wide degree of experiences with and perspectives on these issues, they are meant to further discussion as well as action towards building communities of care.

While I say that this zine was born out of frustration, I must also add that it was nurtured by love. Love for all of those willing to share their stories about illness, love for those who are already taken steps to discuss and improve these (and the many related) issues within their communities, and love for those who will listen to the voices in this zine and then act.

Thanks for reading this zine. Feedback is very welcome: illnesszine@gmail.com. Despite the range of pieces included here, there are many more experiences to share and topics to explore. I'm hoping to create a second issue, so if you're interested in contributing, please be in touch.

Ben
New York City / 2009
illnesszine@gmail.com

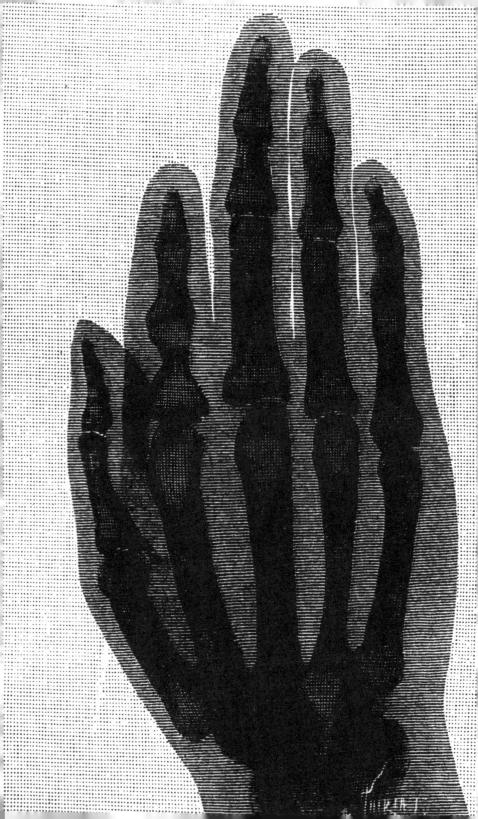

CONTENTS

THANKS

Thanks to everyone who gave this zine their early support and encouragement, especially when I was unsure about the viability of the project and my abilities to complete it. You all really helped to fuel this project.

I sincerely appreciate the efforts of everyone who helped distribute fliers in their towns, while on tour, at their distro tables, as well as those who were willing to post the call on their website and/or through their personal networks.

Thanks to Fly for the amazing illustrations on pages 26, 53, 70 and 86. Check out more of her work at www.peops.org and www.flyspage. com. Thanks also to Kriss of Killer Banshee Studios for the images on 43 and 69.

Thanks to Kat McIntyre not only for being such a good friend but also for her work on *The Worst*, a brilliant zine on death and grief that in no small part helped to inspire my work on this zine.

Carl Williamson not only designed fliers and ads needed throughout the project but also layed out the entire zine. I am so grateful. More than a brilliant designer, he is my very cherished friend.

Thanks to everyone who commented on my articles as well as to those contributors who helped read other pieces when I needed another set of eyes (Brittany, Lizzie, Luci, and Mandy).

Microcosm Publishing rules. I am humbled by—and extraordinarily appreciative of—their support of this project and their decision to publish it.

Extra, extra special thanks to all of the contributors who were willing to share their stories. I am in awe of your bravery and generosity.

Finally, thanks doesn't seem like enough to everyone who supported me when I was sick. All I can say is that I owe you all so, so much. Not only did you help to keep me alive when I was fighting for my life, you also continue to provide the joy and love in my life that makes it worth fighting for. Thanks especially to dad, mom, and Ray who have been there for me in every way imaginable.

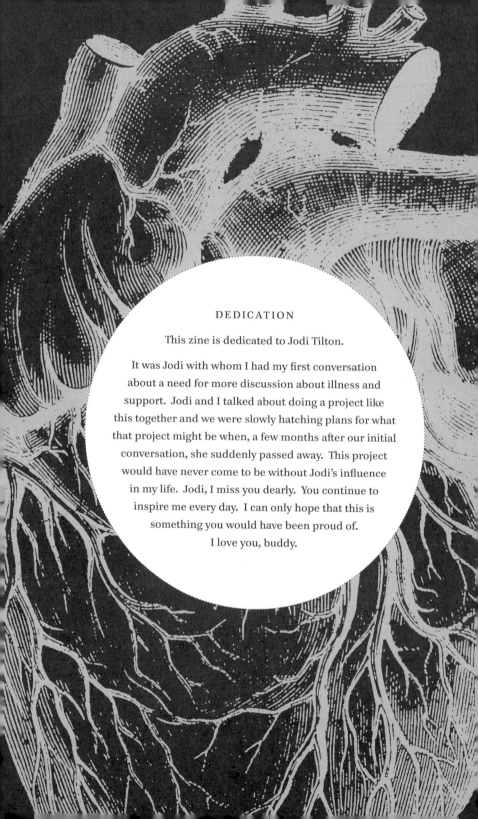

DEDICATION

This zine is dedicated to Jodi Tilton.

It was Jodi with whom I had my first conversation about a need for more discussion about illness and support. Jodi and I talked about doing a project like this together and we were slowly hatching plans for what that project might be when, a few months after our initial conversation, she suddenly passed away. This project would have never come to be without Jodi's influence in my life. Jodi, I miss you dearly. You continue to inspire me every day. I can only hope that this is something you would have been proud of.
I love you, buddy.

NOT OKAY: DEALING WITH INCURABLE ILLNESS

KRISTA CIMINERA

I was diagnosed with Polycystic Kidney Disease two years ago. It is genetic, life threatening, and incurable. The disease comes from my father, with a 50% chance of inheriting it. My brother has it too and so did my aunt.

PKD is a genetic mutation where sometimes, instead of a new kidney cell forming, a cyst forms in its place. These cysts grow over time and end up absorbing the surrounding kidney cells and destroying them. Most people with PKD will have their kidneys fail at some point during their lives. When this happens, the only treatments are dialysis, which is a way of cleaning the blood through the help of a machine, or transplantation.

It was my choice to find out my PKD status. I was asymptomatic at the time and decided that I wanted to find out whether or not I had it. To find out, you need to get a sonogram of your kidneys to determine whether or not there are any cysts.

*   *   *

I am riding my bike to Bellevue Hospital to get a sonogram, up First Avenue on a dirty New York summer day. There is no bicycle parking at the hospital, and in my head I make a bad Jerry Seinfeld-esque joke, something like, "Of course there's no bike parking at the hospital. If you can ride your bike to the hospital, you don't need to be there." Once I am inside the hospital, I find the waiting room and wait to be seen.

The room where I get my sonogram is dim. I enter sheepishly, trying to hold the gown I'm asked to wear closed at the back. There is a small, thin bed alongside the wall, and a woman, the technician, sits next to it in front of a monitor. "Lay down on your side," she says. The lights are off. Grey sunlight comes in sideways through a lone window, stretching and elongating across the walls. And it's dim. Dim like I'm home again and too sick to go to school and my mother is taking care of me. I lay down on the bed, face the wall, and think about my mother coming into check on me while the woman is preparing the machine. She places her hands on my back and begins to rub rhythmically. I imagine it's my mother's hands rubbing my back; the hands that soothed the fever out of me as a child and made the bad things go away. But it is not. It is a stranger in a sterile grey, dead and dull room, looking into a part of me that I could never see. Someone just doing their job.

She does this for a few minutes and then, abruptly, she stops and gets up. "You're done. You can get dressed now," she says, like I've taken part in some sort of seedy exchange. "You'll get the results soon."

She leaves the room, and I'm alone.

*   *   *

My father sits in a recliner in front of a TV with the dialysis machine to his right and a wooden chair between the two. A single window fills the room with cool, fading sunlight, disappearing behind the houses as my father's night on dialysis begins. Two tubes in his right arm connect my father to the machine; one so that his blood can leave, and the other so that it can return. He does this three nights a week, for six hours at a time so that his blood can be cleaned. All of the tubes, blinking lights and locomotion of the machine are for one single purpose: to bring his blood to the thin cylinder that acts as an artificial kidney.

He does this for eight years. I am anywhere from two to ten years old. My sister and I spend a lot of time here, simply called "the dialysis room" which used to be my brother's bedroom before him and my other brother started sharing a room. We make games using the assortment of supplies that can be found here: the blood pressure cuff, the standing scale, the centrifuge. These are our play things and for the moment, while my father waits out another night dependent on this machine, we are oblivious to their meanings.

*   *   *

I'm eight years old and the phone rings as I'm eating dinner in the kitchen with my mom, brothers and sister. Dad is in the dialysis room eating dinner alone. He's on the waiting list to receive a transplant. It's already been a year and a half. Upon the first ring from the phone, my mother tenses, holds her breath, and shoots my brother Greg an awful, menacing look. For the past two weeks, we'd been receiving prank phone calls from the same person. He speaks gibberish, curses and says lewd things, and sometimes says nothing at all. My mother's convinced it's one of my brother's high school friends, since admitting that he and several friends had prank called another friend about a month ago.

It rings several times before she gets up to answer, and she spits out a bitter "Hello" as she holds the receiver to her mouth. She doesn't say anything for a few seconds, she's just listening, and then she explodes screaming, "Why are you doing this? Why are you doing this? Don't you understand that every time the phone rings in this house, I think it's a call from the hospital to tell me that they've found a kidney for my husband? Why are you doing this to us? Just leave us alone, please." She slams the phone onto the hook and collapses, sobbing, onto the countertop. My brothers, sister and I are frozen, backs against our chairs, our eyes wide as we look at each other, at her, and our mouths are open like we're going to say something, but we don't. After a minute, she goes to her bedroom without looking at us.

My brothers, the oldest, seem to know something that I can't understand. My sister and I are scared. None of us says anything. We gather the dirty dishes into the dishwasher and then turn on the TV. Mom doesn't make an appearance for the rest of the night, and our house never receives another prank call again.

*   *   *

I'm ten years old and my parents have just left to go to Boston in a flurry of suitcases and phone calls. They have a kidney for my father. My Aunt Mary, who is my father's sister and got her own transplant a few years before, comes over to take care of us. Apparently, she has been given permission to spoil us for the next week, so we stay home from school, watch rented movies, and eat whipped cream out of the can. I'm happy. Everyone else is happy. And after two weeks, dad comes home. We wait at the window all day, and finally the car drives up. We gather around the door, shouting and jumping, and they walk in, my mother supporting my father. As we run to him my mom puts a hand out and says sternly, "Don't. Be careful. Don't touch him." And I recoil in a kind of fear as they slowly walk the steps to their bedroom, because I've always been able to touch my father before.

*   *   *

I'm fourteen and at the hospital. My father is coming out of a six hour surgery to clip an aneurysm that was found in his brain. The aneurysm is an effect of having PKD, although my parents won't tell us that for many years. Outside of the recovery room, I'm gripping a get well card that I made by hand and had everyone sign. My mom and I are allowed to see him, and he is barely conscious. I hand him the card in his left hand as my mother grips his right. "What's this?" she says without looking at it, and drops the card to the ground. I bend to pick it up and when I stand again, my mother is squeezing his hand with both of hers. Shaking her head with her lips closed tight, she begins to cry and says, "Longest day of my life, Victor. Longest day of my life."

13

I'm sixteen and Aunt Mary is in the hospital because she's feeling pains in her abdomen. My parents say that she'll be fine and out in a few days. But after a few days, my father comes home from the hospital and I can sense that something's wrong. "I don't think she's going to come out of the hospital," he says to us later that night. Her transplanted kidney failed and her body wasn't taking to the dialysis. While she's still conscious, my father asks if she would like to see us, the kids, and she tells him no. "You wouldn't want to see her anyway, not the way she looks now," my father says. And after ten days in the hospital, my aunt, who never had a partner or any children and loved us like her own, dies at the age of fifty four.

*   *   *

It's been almost a month since my sonogram.

"So I have the report right here in front of me," my nephrologist says to me over the phone. "And it looks as though you've got cysts in both your kidneys." I had been sitting lazily in my chair, doodling on a piece of paper, but now I am upright, the pen poised in mid air. I believe I've misheard her and say, "What?"

"You have Polycystic Kidney Disease. Did you know that?" she asks.

"Well, no," I reply. And somehow I stay on the phone for another minute, tell her I will come see her this week, and hang up. I walk out into the living room, and for a moment there is a stillness, like a calm before a storm, like I'm suspended in time, refusing to move forward with this new information. But then, it is upon me and I fall to the ground, the greatest falling down of my life. I am shattered. The glass that separated me from my father's existence is no longer there, and as I clutch my stomach and make painful, sobbing sounds, I am catapulted through memory and meaning. I relive my youth, except I am my father in the dialysis chair as my children crawl around unknowingly, I live in a house that is about to crack under the weight of my fragile mortality, I am in the hospital, I am in the hospital again, and again, and I am dead.

After exhausting myself for an hour I try to find composure so that I can call my parents and tell them that their daughter has a disease.

*   *   *

James Baldwin wrote, "Some people look at you like you've farted when you try to tell them the truth," and I felt the weight of those words as I began to tell people about my diagnosis. It is a topic that stunk up the room with its magnitude and awkwardness. And in an attempt to clear the air, or open a window, many people fell short of what I would call providing positive support. Perhaps because I'm young, because there are no outward symptoms, or just because I am a friend, I suddenly found myself defending the severity of my disease. I am told that I will be okay, that everyone will get sick at some point, and that everyone's going to need health insurance someday. I am reassured that there will be a cure: a thoughtless and meaningless word that resonates in my head like an empty promise.

And I feel powerless. Powerless to explain the complexities of my disease, the feelings that come with the complete and sudden change of my life's narrative, and the guilt I feel in holding onto the anger and fear that feels natural for me at this moment. I feel alone, backed up against the wall and pleading, "Wait, you don't understand." Because how do I begin to describe living with PKD if I am not heard in the first place? How can I begin a discussion of illness if it is dismissed with reassurances before it's even begun?

Not everyone is going to be okay, this is a truth. Only when we accept this truth will we be able to discuss disease in a way that is constructive, helpful, and healing. And in this way, we will be able to expand the ways in which these conversations and interactions can be incorporated into our lives and learn to grow with the people that we wish to care about, instead of apart from them.

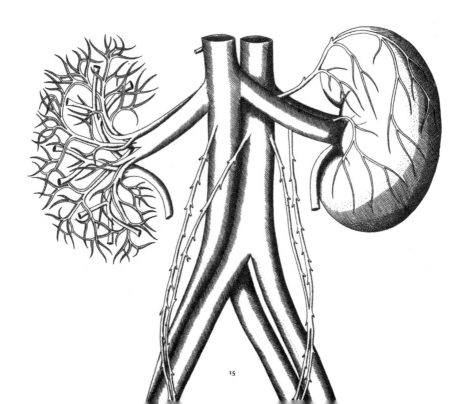

ILLNESS, DISABILITY, AND THE PUNK PARADOX

LUCI

I could feel it again. I was sure of it, that sadly familiar twisting pain in my diaphragm, the crackling when I breathed in – both indications that my lungs were filling with fluid. My swollen ankles molded to the shape of my socks, getting ever tighter as the group I walked with headed to the cemetery to knock back a few beers. I kept walking, laughing, talking, my heart rate reaching highs near 170 beats per minute, my blood pressure low to the point of dizziness and nausea. I didn't say anything, breathing heavily to keep up, because I didn't want to ruin the mood. I thought they wouldn't understand, and I didn't want to lose friends by asking them to accommodate me and my secret: I was living with heart failure.

Born completely healthy, I remained that way until 11 years old, when I developed Idiopathic Dilated Cardiomyopathy. This is a relatively common condition in which the heart loses its ability to pump blood throughout the cardiovascular system, resulting in an enlarged heart and scrappily functioning body. This disease is usually caused by a virus that attacks the heart, but because my disease was diagnosed as "idiopathic" there was no answer to why it had happened to me. In vain I tried to decide what it was I had done that caused my own body to turn against me, while my parents planned the details of a funeral they were told to expect. Four weeks after my diagnosis, I went to the hospital for a surgery to transplant my old heart with a new one. The surgery went smoothly, and I was at home after only 2 weeks of recovery.

Part of living as a transplant recipient is that I have to take immunosuppressive drugs for my entire life. These drugs basically kill my immune system, making it incredibly easy for me to catch any nasty germs that might never bother a person with an immune system. The extreme side effects of my drugs are a constant reminder of my health. I get regular migraines, irregular periods, nausea, I have an incredibly high risk of cancer (I have to be screened at least once a year) and bone density loss makes my back and legs hurt.

It's important to note that my transplant was/is not a cure. It was/is a treatment. I was given a life expectancy of 7-10 years with a chance of survival past that point. For the past year, I've been sick again, the same symptoms of the disease that cost me my first heart. Now, at 21 years old, I am currently living on a kind of life support, a constant intravenous inotrope (a medicine that helps the heart pump more efficiently) that sits inconspicuously in a fanny pack I wear even to bed. As of November 21st, I've been waiting 8 months for a second heart transplant. I am not allowed to be more than 2 hours from my hospital, and clocking in at 2 hours 20 minutes, my current hometown is pushing the limits of how far my rope stretches.

Although this all sounds pretty shitty, I definitely haven't let it stop me in my life. All through high school and into college I involved myself with activism and the punk community, becoming an integral part of several communities, being in bands, making friends, and having fun. In doing these things, I felt like I found a group of people I could belong to that would accept me for who I was, regardless of anything. I didn't ever really talk about my disability because it was something I could easily hide and keep to myself. Some of my friends knew I had a heart transplant years ago, but didn't really know anything about it, so assumed all was well.

Slowly but surely throughout these last 14 months I've lost a place in the community I once had so much faith in. My bandmates didn't understand the fact that I was physically incapable of screaming into a microphone. People I used to hang out with didn't understand why I couldn't ride my bike anymore to their houses or why it was impossible for me to walk anywhere. When I didn't show up to shows, because the venue was smoky or it hurt to stand for a long time, people started dismissing me. For a while I drove my car to do things, but the constant talk of how shitty I was for driving a car really got to me and so eventually I stopped doing even that.

It's been expressed before that I am suspected of utilizing my health problems as a convenience in social situations. People have implied I may be lying about my capabilities or limitations so I can avoid a walk, bike ride, or sexual encounter. I wish people could understand that I don't choose when my disability affects me, and how hurtful it is to not be trusted about such a personal issue.

In what can only be an honest effort to offer help to me, people can become overbearing. Why is it so difficult for me to follow a strict diet? What's so hard about resisting peer pressures? This room/place isn't *that* smoky. It can't be impossible to walk around the block. It would be much more productive if people would *ask* how they can provide support instead of taking it upon themselves to tell me what's in my best interest.

This isn't an uncommon scenario within disabled experience. In everyday life,

When adhering to common cultural norms and behaving within the confines of societal boundaries, disabled people find themselves disguising what ailments they can in order to seem more normal.

In my personal experience, this stands true even more steadfastly in the punk/DIY community. With strong opposition to driving cars, using modern medicine, adhering to common standards of hygiene and living a substance free life, the punk community is quick to ostracize anyone who doesn't live by these means. If a person is physically incapable of riding a bike or walking even a few blocks, which is true sometimes with my illness, they are ridiculed for driving a car instead. If someone has to practice good hygiene in order to avoid complications and infections, or cannot eat potentially harmful food from a dumpster they are immediately judged by that in social circles to mean they aren't as "punk" or "DIY."

It's confusing to me that in a culture that is specifically designed to operate outside the norms of society, how there can be so many rules and guidelines to adhere to. And in a culture that adheres to rules and guidelines that separate people based on their physical abilities, how can a disabled person find allies and support?

Through this past year, my friends have certainly been weeded out from my acquaintances. I have found a core group of people to honestly support me and understand as best they can what I'm going through. Still, the punk community as a whole is not accommodating to people living with illnesses.

The simplest steps can be taken in our individual communities to be more inclusive, but able-bodied folks must realize their privilege before there can be an effort to make our playing grounds more equal. Think about typical activities in your communities and how your level of health determines your participation: Dumpster diving, putting up stencils, shows/venues, and emphasis on alternative means of transportation.The ability to run away if detected, to stand for long periods of time, to be resistant to viruses and disease, and to ride a bike or walk somewhere are all examples that require some level of physical ability and fitness. It's not that people with disabilities love using gas, are lazy, or are hypochondriacs-we want the same things, why else would we be involved in this community?

If there is a house/venue where people hang out all the time, why not make that house smoke-free? It's healthier for everyone, and makes that environment at least an option to people not able to breathe in secondhand smoke.

At community dinners, and in collective houses, people could label food as being dumpstered. This would help those who need to be more conscious about what they're eating know about potentially harmful bacteria.

When there is a show, be aware of the dynamic at the front of the room. Is there an overly aggressive mosh pit going on? Observe the kind of people standing at the back of the room. Do people with illnesses/disabilities (or just people who don't want to be pushed to the floor) deserve to be in the back? Challenge the common thought that the only way to enjoy a show is to be violent.

Are you quick to judge a person based on the visibility of dirt/smell or lack thereof? Writing this seems silly, but it's true that in punk/DIY circles, if someone is clean or not visibly disheveled, there can be serious misconceptions abound. Think about how being dirty can mean being sick for someone with a lowered immune system. Be aware of your surroundings when you are sick with a cold/flu, let people know you are ill, so someone doesn't make the mistake of exposing themselves if they shouldn't.

Individually, think about your personal hygiene when having sex with an ill/disabled person (actually in general). Have you been tested recently? Do your fingernails have dirt under them? For someone with no immune system or who is on certain prescription drugs, simple S.T.I's or vaginal infections can easily become fatal.

What kind of words do you use without consideration about their meaning? Using "retarded" or "lame" as insults is just as disempowering to disabled people as using "pussy" or "cunt" as insults is to female anatomy and should be avoided the same.

How many people in your community are open about having disabilities or an illness? If there is no one, do you think it's because someone is afraid of coming out? Why or why not? What is your community doing to make these people feel welcome, equal, and included?

I live in a communal house with 8 roommates. Everyone I share my home with has been great about maintaining an open dialogue about what things could make me more comfortable/less likely to continue getting sick. For example, we had our ducts cleaned out this winter before turning on the heat because of the risk of mold exposure. Also, people label dumpstered foods in the fridge, thoroughly clean dishes, wash their hands after going to the bathroom/doing other stuff, and let me know if they are sick.

If more people become actively involved in these and other processes, disabled/ill folks can begin to feel more comfortable and safe. With more people in our circles being offered a voice, there's no telling what we can accomplish.

SCAR MATES

RAINBOW

He and I sat on his dorm room bed gazing into each other's eyes. Contentment swelled within my chest; maybe I could let my guard down. I let him lean close to me, his hand wandering underneath my t-shirt. He began lifting my shirt. I gasped, hesitant to let him see what I had only casually mentioned: scars scoring my abdomen, reminders of the surgeries which had saved my life.

A shocked "hmm!" escaped his lips as he examined my body. He let my shirt fall back down into place and we began kissing. "Maybe he'd forget about my stomach if we went further," I thought. Yet, I knew that I deserved a proper boyfriend, not just fooling around. He would have to get to know me better, even love me, before I'd let him do anything else. We just kissed.

We cuddled and watched television for another couple hours and then he drove me home. "We should do this again sometime," I said.

"Sure, definitely," he replied. We kissed briefly before he left.

The next time we talked he was aloof. He wasn't as talkative as usual, which worried me. (I liked him. Did he like me?) "So, when would you like to meet up again?" I asked cautiously.

"I don't know..." he began. "I'm kinda busy this week."

"Oh. Whenever you're free is fine," I replied, instantly knowing he could sense my desperation.

"No offense, but I just don't see this going anywhere," he said bluntly. "I'm definitely attracted to your mind... just, uh, not... to your body. I'm sorry."

"It's my scars, right?" I retorted.

"Yeah... they're just too weird," he replied. "I really am sorry."

"I guess they wouldn't look so bad if I weren't chubby, huh?" I asked spitefully.

"Uh, I guess... they just freak me out... I'm sorry," he said. "We can still talk if you want."

I knew that he didn't mean to hurt me, but I cried for hours after that, wanting to rip off my fat rolls and burn away my scars. The pain of open heart surgery and a kidney transplant combined didn't even touch the emotional pain of rejection. Not only that, but his attitude reminded me of every other guy I had been interested in. They simply insisted that I cover myself, that I be ashamed because they couldn't be bothered to see the other things that make me beautiful.

A week later I decided to browse a dating website on which I had a profile. I noticed that someone had taken my compatibility test and scored rather low. They were still online, so I took a chance and decided to instant message them.

He quickly issued me a warning: "I'm disgusting," he typed.

"Why?" I asked.

"I cough up phlegm all day, and shit fat," he replied. "I have cystic fibrosis."

"Oh, yeah?" I typed, intrigued by his honesty. "I can piss out of my navel... with a catheter."

We chatted all night. I told him about my premature birth, my eye surgeries, and my open heart surgery to fix a defect which would have killed me. I told him about how I couldn't drain my bladder completely when I was a child, so my doctor had used my appendix as a conduit from my navel to my bladder, allowing me to drain the excess urine. I told him how despite catheterizing myself daily, my kidneys had failed from the reflux by age 11, prompting me to have a kidney transplant.

He explained how his disease had mucked up his lungs with mucus, making them havens for bacteria. He told me how he had to use a nebulizer twice daily in order to deliver antibiotics and saline to his lungs. In addition, he had a hard time absorbing fat from food, so he stayed underweight. Enzymes helped him digest his meals. Also, he was diabetic from mucus building up in his pancreas. His abdomen bore scars from a feeding tube and other surgeries.

Surprisingly, we had much more in common than our respective illnesses. Soon we met in person, quickly falling in love. The first time he saw my scars, he kissed each one, then looked into my eyes. "They're beautiful," he said. A year and a half later, we are still together. He makes me appreciate my second chance at life, and I help him cope with the daily realities of CF. Most of all, we remind each other that we are not our illnesses. We are people. We are fighters. We can make a life together.

BLACK CLOUD

EMIKO BADILLO

This black cloud over my head. I fight it everyday and every moment of my life until I die. It's an incurable disease, and it nearly ruined me. My curse. My nemesis. My lifelong companion.

It's called End Stage Renal Disease, but most know it as kidney disease. This came to me out of the blue when I was 28 years old and just beginning to be comfortable in my own skin.

My life up until the sickness seemed filled with trouble and chaos, and it took me almost three decades to stop low-self-esteem-fueled behaviors and start liking myself. With the help of my husband, Chad, I was happy and looking forward to our future in Portland, Oregon. We just opened a small vegan grocery store and were excited about so many new possibilities. So with all that positive eagerness in our lives, my sudden illness seemed even more vicious and tragic. The biggest joke ever played.

It seemed like one day I was healthy, the next day not, and my symptoms were swift and severe. It started with migraines. Never even having slight headaches my whole life, teeth chattering migraines out of the blue was scary.

Being new to town, I went to a naturopath my friend had seen before, and she made the situation even more desperate. Misdiagnosing me as having a "virus," she said my blood pressure seemed "a little high" and claimed my vegan diet might be in need of some changing. She prescribed a ton of supplements I can't even remember and told me to keep drinking chamomile tea. Ironically, when you have kidney failure, drinking a lot of fluids is one of the last things you should do. I just got worse and worse.

Blindness was next. Unknowingly my blood pressure had shot up so fast that it hemorrhaged my retinas, and blind spots started growing in my eyes until I could hardly see anything but a dark mist. Looking these symptoms up online didn't help either because it named every illness but kidney failure.

Nausea, puking, trapped fluid in my lungs and body, and muscle atrophy quickly followed. Little did I know this was the domino effect from my kidneys kicking the bucket to the poisoning and breakdown of my body. What was worse, the physical crippling or the not knowing why this was happening?

These were bad, bad times. Chad was going insane with stress and worry, taking care of me and working our new store by himself. I was choking on the fluid in my lungs when I tried to sleep, threw up what little I ate, and I could hardly even walk anymore. We didn't have any close friends yet, no support system except each other, so I eventually had to reach out further for help and called my mom. She flew from Texas the next day.

I saw an eye doctor a couple weeks prior who referred me to a retinal specialist. My mom escorted me to my appointment, and I was practically crawling and semi-conscious by that point. The doctor could tell right away something was wrong, and right away he checked my blood pressure. Before I knew it I was in the intensive care unit being hooked to blood pressure lowering IVs. I had kidney failure. What a surprise. Never crossed my mind that was the cause of my months of misery.

I woke up in ICU the next day stabilized and tired. My pain was suddenly wiped clean. This complete relief from the agony of dying and unknowing somehow made everything the doctors and nurses told me less grave. I had End Stage Renal Disease. That is a complete failure of my kidneys, the organs that help you pee and excrete toxins from your blood. Essential to staying alive. Kidney disease doesn't run in my family; I didn't have any other health issues before. To this day we still don't know why my kidneys died.

The first week in the hospital I was bombarded with so much bad news, yet I seemed happy and upbeat. Everyone saw it as me being a strong woman, but it wasn't that. It's because my symptoms prior were so, so horrible, I thought to myself, as long as I never had to go through that level of suffering again, I could take whatever they had to give me. Dialysis for the rest of my life? Fine. Kidney transplant? Fine. Lots of medicines with side effects? Fine.

There is no cure for this disease. We ESRDers have a few options: dialysis, transplant, or death. Now that I've done the first two and almost the last, I can say that having a transplant has been the best way for me to keep anything near the same lifestyle I had before. I did both forms of dialysis. Hemodialysis, the most familiar one, I did for a month. I went to a clinic 3 times a week for 4 hours and got hooked up to a machine that cleaned the toxins from my blood. I was the youngest at the clinic, and trying to drown out the constant complaining and sexism from my sick neighbors, I'd put on my headphones and try to ignore them. I always left there sad and hopeless.

Peritoneal dialysis was a relief because I did this myself in the privacy of my home. It's not as common of a therapy because, having a disease that normally plagues older folks, they usually don't have the dexterity to fulfill the rather rigorous regimen. I filled and drained saline into and out of my peritoneal cavity 3 times a day through a tube that was implanted into my stomach. Sounds grody, but this gave me more freedom, and I performed this on myself for nearly a year until my transplant. I could even take my supplies with me and do it anywhere I wanted (within clean-reason), which meant I could travel again and adjust my dialysis according to my own schedule.

In general with dialysis, you're usually tired and nauseous, you have more restrictions with what you eat (salt salt salt), but food doesn't taste good anyway. Most looming is your life expectancy. Not so optimistic. This makes that black cloud bigger and darker...with thunder and lightning.

At first I was content on the thought of dialysis for the rest of my life. My doctors were pushing transplant right away, but after what I went through, I wasn't up for the trials and tribulations of having major surgery. Also, not having a true idea of what dialysis puts one through, I thought I could live a long, full life that way. When I found out life expectancy with diaysis is 10–30 years, I freaked. My expectations of growing old with Chad were suddenly compromised, and I realized why my doctors wanted me to go under the knife so bad. A younger person with a good matching kidney could live out a relatively normal and lengthy life. There was no question my brothers would get tested first because my family is so supportive, and any one of us would be willing to risk our lives to save each other. So, after a pretty quick pre-screening process, a year to the day of being diagnosed, I received my brother, Brian's kidney, and it's been a great match.

Now, with my transplant, all I do is take my medicine, go to my doctor appointments, and keep an eye on myself. I can eat whatever I want, go wherever I want, do whatever activity I want (except probably anything that might get me punched in the stomach). It's like I've been reborn, and I forget a little more everyday what dialysis was like... generally. Of course, there's way more to it than that.

Sickness isn't a subject people enjoy discussing or hearing about. It's a mortal reminder for both sides, but it's there, and sometimes it's happening to the most unlikely people. When you're young and given a short life expectancy, sometimes it's hard not to want to give up. Life almost left me, and my initial joy of overcoming death was quickly taken over by fragility and confusion. Why, why, why? Unanswerable questions were taking over. Sometimes there's only so much loved ones can do for you until you need professional help. I can honestly say my therapist saved my life in that first crucial year.

It's been better since my transplant. The memory of dialysis is slowly fading day by day, good or bad. But when you're dealing with something negative that is never going to leave your side, how can you not let it get you down from time to time?

I'm pretty sure I can speak for my fellow sickies and say having an illness is more than a bummer. If I stop too long to think about my disease and mortality, I can cry no sweat. Being sick isn't something I will ever get used to. No one would guess from seeing me how rotted I am inside. My health is that of a 80 year old, but on the outside I seem to be a happy-go-lucky 33. And that's the way I want it. I want to be like my peers or whomever I would've been if I never got sick. When I meet someone new there's always that tension in my head of when or if I should tell this new person what lurks inside me. It's something so important to me, yet you always have to wait for the right time to tell your new friend, "oh by the way…" The last thing I want is pity and attention, but I always know sooner or later I'll have to talk about it, and I feel like the image one might have had of me will be stained. It's not that I'm ashamed, but it's complex. I don't feel like everyone else, but I try to. I want to educate people about living with an illness, but I don't want to be treated differently. Yet I'm not like everyone else and I have to be treated differently sometimes.

From talking with other younger sick people, we are almost secretive about our illnesses mainly because we don't want to be a burden, and we don't want charity. I find myself hiding my medicines down below the table when I'm eating a meal with friends, and I have to take them. We still want to seem strong and bulletproof, and this makes us keep our heartaches on the inside. Torturing ourselves with our self-prejudice and pain. For me, the funny and hypocritical part about it all is, since I do keep it to myself so much, sometimes when I'm not feeling my best and do want comfort or sympathy, most people don't remember right away that I'm sick, and I'm left to keep dealing alone. But that's actually okay for me. I would rather have people forget I'm sick than worry. This probably hasn't been the most therapeutically positive way for me to take my sickness, but it's my own natural survival instinct I can't control.

Even after five years of living with this, I still have those feelings of despair of fear of death, and it is so hard to keep my head up when the feeling falls over me. I have small memories of what I used to be like, but I can hardly remember anymore who that was. This is me now, and it's hard, but at the same time it's hard not to want to keep fighting and making your time the best possible. There's really no other choice. I believe that strength to survive is in all of us.

I was once young and healthy, too. It was the best. Now that I am what I am, I hate to think of what I could have done to maybe make life a little easier now. Isn't it always a case of "if I knew then what I know now?" My hopes from writing this are that maybe one person reading will really, truly hear and understand.

Some illnesses can be prevented or minimized with early detection. Most of us don't have health insurance, but sometimes something as simple as a blood test can catch a problem before you see any signs or symptoms. And it should be mandatory to learn about your family's health history. If you know something runs in your family, get checked for it. Instead of saving up for records or tattoos, get a physical. Splurge on your health. Not as fun, but more significant, and you only need one a year to be safe. Of course when you're young, health never seems important until you get sick, but it's never too late to start caring. It happened to me. It can happen to you. It's happened to a lot of us already. Have fun, be free, be happy, but also take care. We are not as invincible as we think.

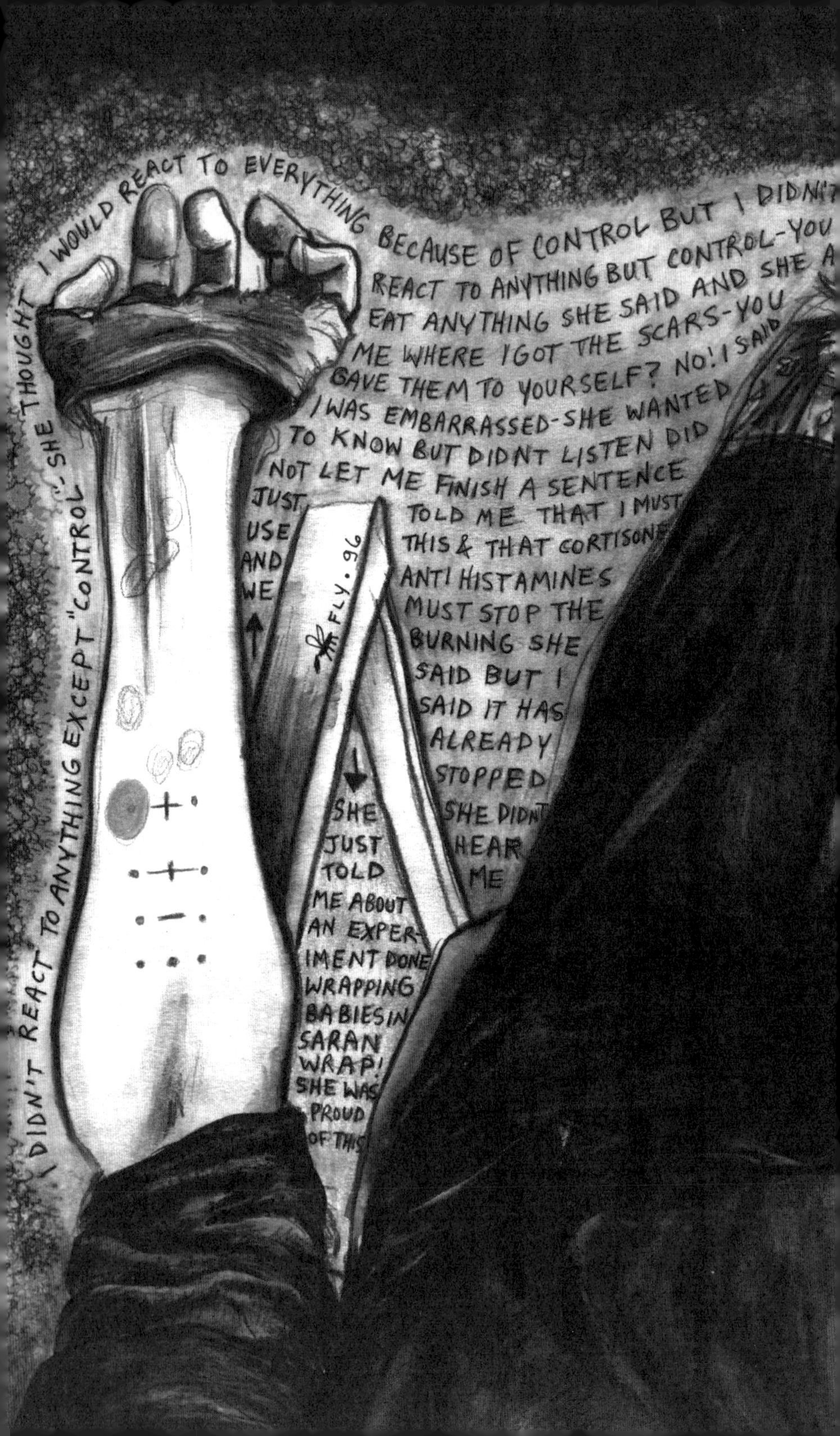

I DIDN'T REACT TO ANYTHING EXCEPT "CONTROL"- SHE THOUGHT I WOULD REACT TO EVERYTHING
BECAUSE OF CONTROL BUT I DIDN'T
REACT TO ANYTHING BUT CONTROL-YOU
EAT ANYTHING SHE SAID AND SHE A
ME WHERE I GOT THE SCARS-YOU
GAVE THEM TO YOURSELF? NO! I SAID
I WAS EMBARRASSED-SHE WANTED
TO KNOW BUT DIDNT LISTEN DID
NOT LET ME FINISH A SENTENCE
JUST USE AND WE
TOLD ME THAT I MUST
THIS & THAT CORTISONE
ANTI HISTAMINES
MUST STOP THE
BURNING SHE
SAID BUT I
SAID IT HAS
ALREADY
STOPPED
SHE DIDNT
HEAR
ME
SHE JUST TOLD ME ABOUT AN EXPERIMENT DONE WRAPPING BABIES IN SARAN WRAP! SHE WAS PROUD OF THIS
FLY. 96

THE INVISIBLE WITNESS

EMILY KLAMER

As a person living with degenerative disc disease (DDD), scoliosis, and supraventricular tachycardia (SVT), my curvatures, arrhythmias, and disintegrations have been mapped out, illuminated, diagnosed, and cemented in both my medical records and self-identity. While I've been living with scoliosis and SVT (a heart rhythm disorder caused by an extra electrical pathway in my heart, like a short circuit) ever since I was in grade school, an acute episode of sudden excruciating back pain in January of 2007 that left me unable to stand or sit up for days catapulted me into the world of constantly navigating the medical system and living with chronic pain and spinal instability. While these physical problems have increasingly become more salient features of my identity over the past couple of years, because my illnesses/disabilities are invisible and my body appears to be healthy and able (most of the time), I struggle with negotiating the practice of self-identification. Since I don't fit into the prototypical mold of what disability has been constructed to mean in this culture and because I can "pass" as an able bodied person, I often feel unworthy identifying as dis/abled.

Furthermore, degenerative disc disease is a misnomer. DDD isn't actually a disease; it is a condition in which the jelly-like, fluid-filled discs in between the vertebrae break down. It is even seen as a normal repercussion of aging, a type of "ordinary" disability. Yet, diagnosed at 18, the DDD eating away at my spine can be seen as quite the oddity. I am always the youngest person in my orthopedist's waiting room, and the disbelieving chorus of "But you're too *young!*" haunts my medical visits and experience of living with DDD. My prematurely geriatric spine acts as a harbinger of the processes that constrain and plague the body as it ages. Seen as ordinary among the elderly, degenerative disc disease functions as an extraordinary anomaly among the young.

My body consequently embodies the lurking threat of illness and disability that is so feared in our culture. In a culture that attempts to obsessively control our bodies, ill and dis/abled bodies represent an unruly deviation from the norm. Our ill and dis/abled bodies are literal embodiments of our culture's insecurity regarding the mortality and imperfectness of the human body, and are therefore hidden and rendered "private" matters. Ill and dis/abled bodies also disturb the western and capitalistic value of the self-sufficient, autonomous, productive body, and are therefore relegated to the margins of society, our inhabited transgressions smothered and stigmatized.

I feel as if I occupy a liminal space along the continuum of ability and well/illness. While my body appears to be able and healthy, living with my multiple diagnoses has required constant negotiation and treatment. Due to their invisibility, it's hard for me to feel validated about the extent to which my chronic back pain and lurking threat of an SVT episode, during which my heart rate skyrockets up to 250 beats a minute and my chest becomes so tight I need to sit down, have changed my life and self-identity. Nowadays, even the most mundane routines (such as grocery shopping and sitting through class) are undertaken with a vigilant self-consciousness. I have become increasingly aware of how our society and its structures are constructed according to a bodily norm (healthy, young, non-disabled, male) that most of us don't, or will not, fit into at some point in our lives. Straddling both sides of the ability/wellness continuum, I now operate from a standpoint that allows me to see a wide spectrum of ability. I was forced to acknowledge how fleeting ability and good health can be, and therefore how dangerous disability and illness are perceived by a culture that seeks to discipline and contain the body and all of its unruly messes, dysfunction, and decline.

The experience of illness and/or disability can be likened to a body of water most of us will be submerged within, either as the sick or the caretaker, at one point or another. As Wendell writes in her work, *The Rejected Body*, "Unless we die suddenly, we are all disabled eventually." Some of us are only temporarily dunked into the depths, while others will bob among the crests and troughs for our entire lives. Either way, the majority of us end up wet eventually. This impending shared experience can be used as a point of departure for temporarily abled bodied people to work towards a more viable solidarity with sick/dis/abled people. As Wendell also notes "Realizing that aging is disabling helps non-disabled people to see that people with disabilities are not 'Other,' that they are really themselves at a later time."

When able-bodied/well people acknowledge their own tenuous grip on the states of health and temporary ability, those struggling to keep their heads above water won't have to struggle so hard to keep afloat. Recognizing our shared commonality is crucial in order to bear witness to each other, to craft communities that are accountable to all of our different abilities. People living with illness and dis/ability need spaces in which our voices can be heard and our bodies recognized. We need spaces in which our complicated narratives can be shared, validated, and heard. In our social justice and radical struggles, abilities related to health and the body must be taken into account just as much as race, class, sex, gender, sexuality, and nation in the fight against multiple systems of domination.

"A LETTER TO FAMILY & FRIENDS WITHOUT HEPATITIS"

SARAH HUGHES

My dad battled chronic Hepatitis C for five years. He wrote the following letter three months before his first coma that sent him in and out of hospitals for six months, eventually leading up to his final breath.

At the time he sent this letter - May of 2004 - to us, he was relatively fine; but what does a word like 'fine' mean four years into a chronic condition like cirrhosis of the liver? His body began deteriorating shortly after his diagnosis and attempt of treatment in 1999. He could not stay on the treatment, as his illness was far too advanced, and his body could not handle the medication in such a way that would allow him to deal with his life. Chronic illness is expensive. With such great insurance and supportive, understanding employment, he contin- ued working and quit the treatments. The first apparent physical deteriora- tion began in November of 2000. His teeth slowly fell out, a side effect of his interferon treatments. So began his body's steady decline. Then the HCV began its course. Nothing prepared me for the more permanent, physical ways his disease would act on his body. When he lost his teeth, he just got dentures. But there were symptoms that could not be easily covered up in this way. Shortly after his teeth, his belly expanded and hardened, as fluid accumulated in his abdomen. The lean man I had known for eighteen years of my life was forever altered. By 2003 his lower legs swelled, turned purplish, and developed open sores from a kind of diabetes that comes with liver disease. These developments in his illness were always horrifying at first, and then with time it just seemed normal, like it had always been that way. He continued to drive to work each day, drive home each day, nap each day, and live with it all each day. Austin Against War was a local activist group he participated in, proudly displaying his signs in the yard. Some weekends my dad would pack sandwiches for like-minded, fel- low members from that group, as they set out to rally at local Wal-Marts, handing out information about how the community was being negatively impacted by a myriad of issues. You could also find him buying nose spray and hard candies at Wal-Mart. My dad was funny that way, set in his ways, but also always wanting to fight the good fight, or help anyone in need.

Hepatitis C, commonly referred to as HCV, is spread by blood-to-blood contact. Once infected, 15-40% of people clear the virus from their system. The remaining 60-85% go on to develop chronic HCV (more than six months of infection) that usually leads to cirrhosis of the liver and liver cancer. Most people progress to cirrhosis within twenty-thirty years, often with few to no symptoms before then. Most symptoms do not become prevalent until there is significant scarring of the liver. Testing went into effect in 1992, and finding HCV early, before much scarring, usually leads to a much better interaction with the drugs available for treatment. Chronic HCV can lead to swollen abdomen along with abdominal pain from fluid retention, bone pain, jaundice, enlarged veins, extreme fatigue, nausea, depression, cognitive changes, flu-like symptoms, inflammation of the kidneys, diabetes, and on and on. It is a chronic illness, and the pain is ongoing.

Even though my dad continued living his life much like before his diagnosis, these symptoms inflicted him day to day, whether we thought about it or not. Luckier than some, he had a supportive doctor who helped him manage his pain and depression. My mom was very unsupportive of him, ashamed of his illness. While my sister and I were never short of love and support, I know it was deeply painful for him to not have a supportive partner during the final years. In many ways this letter was for her, and sadly she dismissed it, as she did with too much of his pain and suffering. Additionally, this letter was a way to express to his daughters that his pain was always present and I think he needed us to understand that at this time, to understand the constant battle he was in day in and day out. I think he just needed us not to forget this battle as we all went about our lives. In many ways, he could not go about his life, not like he did before. Each day was a struggle, at times, even each hour.

A LETTER TO FAMILY & FRIENDS WITHOUT HEPATITIS—THIS ONE TO FAMILY

Dear Precious Dysfunctional Family:

Having Hepatitis means many things change, and a lot of them are invisible. Unlike having cancer or being hurt in an accident, most people do not understand even a little about HCV and its effects, and of those that think they know, many are actually misinformed. In the spirit of informing those who wish to understand …These are the things that I would like to you to understand about me before you judge me… Please understand that being sick doesn't mean I'm not still a human being. I have to spend most of my day in considerable pain and exhaustion, and if you visit I probably don't seem like much fun to be with, but I'm still me stuck inside this body. I still worry about life and work and my family and friends, and most of the time

I'd still like to hear you talk about yours too.

Please understand the difference between "happy" and "healthy." When you've got the flu you probably feel miserable with it, but I've been sick for years. I can't be miserable all the time, in fact I work hard at not being miserable. So if you're talking to me and I sound happy, it means I'm happy. That's all. It doesn't mean that I'm not in a lot of pain, or extremely tired, or that I'm getting better, or any of those things. Please don't say, "Oh, you're sounding better!" I am not sounding better. I am sounding happy. If you want to comment on that, you're welcome.

Please understand that being able to stand up for ten minutes doesn't necessarily mean that I can stand up for twenty minutes, or an hour. And just because I managed to stand up for thirty minutes yesterday doesn't mean that I can do the same today. With a lot of diseases you're either paralyzed, or you can move. With this one it gets more confusing.

Please repeat the above paragraph substituting "sitting," "walking," "thinking," "being sociable," and so on...it applies to everything. That's what Hepatitis does to you. Please understand that HCV is variable. It's quite possible (for me, it's common) that one day I am able to walk Sissy around the block, while the next day I'll have trouble getting to the kitchen. Please don't attack me when I'm ill by saying, "But you did it before!" If you want me to do something then ask if I can. In a similar vein, I may need to cancel an invitation at the last minute, if this happens please do not take it personally. Please understand that "getting out and doing things" does not make me feel better. Telling me that I need a treadmill, or that I just need to loose (or gain) weight, get this exercise machine, join this gym, try these classes... may frustrate me to tears, and is not correct...if I was capable of doing these things, don't you know that I would? I am working with my doctor and physical therapist and am already doing the exercise and diet that I am supposed to do. Another statement that hurts is, "You just need to push yourself more, exercise harder..." Obviously HCV deals directly with muscles, and because our muscles don't repair themselves the way your muscles do, this does far more damage than good and could result in recovery time in days or weeks or months from a single activity. Also, Hepatitis may cause secondary depression (wouldn't you get depressed if you were hurting and exhausted for years on end!?!) but it is not created by depression. Please understand that if I say I have to sit down/lie down/take these pills now, that I do have to do it right now—it can't be put off or forgotten just because I'm out for the day (or whatever). **Hepatitis does not forgive.**

If you want to suggest a cure to me, don't. It's not because I don't appreciate the thought, and it's not because I don't want to get well. It's because I have had almost every single one of my friends suggest one at one point or another. At first I tried them all, but then I realized that I was using up so much energy trying things that I was making myself sicker, not better. If there was something that cured, or even helped, all people with Hepatitis then we'd know about it. This is not a drug-company conspiracy, there is worldwide networking (both on and off the Internet) between people with Hepatitis if something worked we would KNOW.

If after reading that, you still want to suggest a cure, then do it, but don't expect me to rush out and try it. I'll take what you said and discuss it with my doctor.

In many ways I depend on you…people who are not sick – I need you to visit me when I am too sick to go out… Sometimes I need you to help me with shopping, cooking or cleaning (mowing, raking, or cleaning out flower beds would be nice… LOL). I may need you to take me to the doctor, or to the physical therapist (most likely pick me up… Ha!) I need you on a different level too…you're my link to the outside world… if you don't come visit me, then I might not get to see you… and, as much as it's possible, I need you to understand me. Take Care.

Peace & Love

Moi

Austin, TX

May, 2004

A DAUGHTER'S REFLECTION

My dad used to sign his emails and cards "Moi" as a funny, sentimental name. He was sarcastic, a jokester, but also had a very sentimental way about him, always finding unique and subtle ways to express his love and affection. After the letter, I felt an overwhelming sense of understanding and appreciation of his constant struggle to manage his pain, his depression, and to go on fighting. For a moment, I conceptualized what it might be like, this constant pain and suffering, and how one would learn to deal with that in order to go out into each day as they once did. This was coupled with rage toward my mom who would not express this understanding. Even those closest to someone suffering from a chronic illness can lose sight of their constant pain, as it is extremely difficult to care for someone through chronic illness, slowly spiraling into worse and more horrifying symptoms. My dad often spoke of people in his HCV support group who lost contact with family members due to their illness, and this was an ongoing fear he harbored and often spoke about to me. Almost angry with him, I could not comprehend how he did not know that my love and support would always be with him. But I also know that much of this fear originated from the lack of support he received from my mom.

One complication of caring for a parent with a chronic illness is how you can interpret certain behaviors as selfish or too needy, because they are so consumed with their illness. At times, I remember feeling my dad was not interested in my day-to-day life, because he would express jealousy of the time I spent with friends, away from him. After the letter, I realized my dad did try and meet me in my life. Some days, on his way home from work, he would stop by for a short visit, rest a bit, talk a bit, and then be on his way. I love these small captures of time I carry with me. I realized these visits were a way for him to express his appreciation, his need and love for me. Going to Goodwill to shop for an old pair of Levis, catching a movie, coming over to take his dog on a walk, or coming over to sit and just be around were some ways I met him in his life. In many ways, my life was going on and his life was slowly ending, and this letter put that in perspective. He was not selfish, but scared. My sister and I continued to love and support him, to attempt to ease his and our fear. As for my dad, he went about his life as usual. I think he said his piece, and just wanted to remind us that he was in a struggle for his life, and it was a painful struggle. To someone on the outside, you may think how would you not be reminded that he was so sick with his swollen belly, legs, sores, fake teeth, fatigue. A person can get used to almost anything. In living your life, it is important for a caregiver to try and maintain some perspective on how a loved one is in constant pain and struggle. They need you to understand, to remember, to acknowledge their fight. As I read my dad's letter now, it seems to say, "Don't forget this battle I have fought...it was for you, too, that I fought... don't forget me."

I never forgot, and I never will. You were brave. Your fight was for you and for us.

IT HURTS.
NO REALLY.
IT HURTS!

JOE BIEL

In late 2008 I was diagnosed with Hypoglycemia after more than fifteen years of dealing with its symptoms: falling asleep without notice, being underweight, having trouble focusing, bad gas, ravenous hunger, joint pain, locked muscles, experiencing painful digestion, memory loss, long-term destruction of my thyroid and adrenal gland, brain damage, and eventually hitting the low where I really couldn't function on a day to day basis.

Hypoglycemia is basically your body not producing enough glucose for your blood. That's why it's called low blood sugar. This means that your body will sometimes send more blood into your brain to increase your glucose levels, which normally results in a migraine, or more commonly non-essential parts of the nervous system are shut down as your blood sugar drops, causing mood swings, personality changes, fatigue, circulatory changes, depression, wear on the thyroid, pituitary, and adrenal gland, anxiety, and in extreme cases eventually passing out or even death.

Decreased glucose to the brain flows less oxygen to important parts of your brain, which makes it hard to focus, perform basic functions, and in the long term causes neurotic behavior, personality changes, and even psychosis. Virtually all clinically psychotic people qualify as low blood sugar (what we don't know is if the chicken comes before the egg or vice versa).

Your endocrine system, particularly the adrenal gland, tries to pick up the slack but over many years wears out. This is the theory of why I fall asleep unpredictably and suddenly. My adrenal gland is worn out and cannot function when it is needed. My case is extreme enough that I need to eat foods that are high in fat and protein every hour or so and I need to categorically avoid sugars and carbs. So it's like the vegan Adkins diet in practice.

But everything I've described above hasn't been the worst part of it.

It's much harder to handle when your so-called progressive radical punk community doesn't know how to interact with you and your problems.

At the time of my low my partner was also experiencing her own physical problems and had withdrawn from communities that she was once very active in, in part because of her health.

With both of us being in pain and socially withdrawn, it allowed me to see how punk communities interact with sick people: by ignoring them.

There are and were many well-intentioned individuals who sincerely wanted to help but just didn't know what to do. I certainly give credit for effort but the whole experience just made me feel like there is yet another gaping hole in the way our "progressive" community is uneducated and not stepping up.

The problem is further compounded if you are undiagnosed or don't have a name for your combination of symptoms (read: "it's all in her head"). If there's one thing that you take from this, believe your peers when they tell you that they hurt or are sick. Visit them and hang out with them even when they are low functioning. I've seen this problem play out over and over. You get sick, you get forgotten.

So then the obvious conclusion is to listen to your friends and peers, believe them, and offer them the kind of support they are looking for. It's stupid to say things like "this is what you should do" or "have you considered that it's all in your head?" because, believe it or not, they have very likely researched it much more than you have and already worried heavily about the latter. They don't need to hear it from you, who just comes across as doubting. Sympathy (e.g. "that sucks" or "I'm sorry") is a better place to start. Everybody is different too so talk to them and see what they need from you.

Even as I've gotten my diet and medication under control and have reassumed a more functional life, I still feel a bit left in the dust by my people. I grew up with very strong ideas about punk and its interconnected politics. It was the family that I wasn't raised with; the one that actually cared about my well-being. Certainly, I have failed it and taking care of the well-being of others at times, but this problem seemed more systemic. No volume of good intentions could solve this problem. It would require educational materials like this zine to really make people understand.

ME AND MY BROTHER

RACHEL

I confess: I was not always the best big sister. For starters, when my dad brought me to the hospital at age two I was initially filled with excitement. I chatted and giggled on our drive over, eager to see the new human being that was now my sibling. However, my excitement quickly faded and turned to disappointment as my dad pointed my brother out to me behind the glass wall. "That one? That is my baby brother??" I asked with some shock, "but I want the one with the red hair!"

A year or so later, in my three-year-old wisdom, I tried to give my brother away. I called the operator (having been told this is what you do when you have a problem) and explained that my brother really needed to go. This event was followed by many instances of pinching, scratching, and hair pulling throughout our years growing up. Not surprisingly, the more-often-than-not end result was my brother crying and me being punished. Of course, this only made me dislike him more, and led to future instances of pinching, scratching, biting and hair pulling.

In spite of all of this, as far back as I can remember, if there was any situation in which I could protect or stand up for my brother, I would. When the neighbor down the street who was probably a foot taller than me and a foot and a half taller than my brother was picking on him, I came to his defense, yelling at the bully to stop. "Who is going to make me?" he asked. "ME!!!" I yelled, "Because I am his big sister!!!" Whatever dislike I had towards him in our younger years passed as we grew, and he became one of my closest friends. The strong sense of needing to protect and support him in whatever situation I could has never faded.

Like other siblings close together in age, my brother and I developed a way of communicating with one another without words. As far back as I can remember glances we shared or faces we made to one another expressed our thoughts far better than words might have. I used to joke that my brother and I could even communicate telepathically and through our dreams.

When I got the news that my brother had cancer, the first thing I wanted to do was to put myself in his place. "Why him? It should be me instead." It was incredibly painful to feel that there was no way that I could protect him from this illness and everything that accompanied it. From this point forward, I felt I was being served a daily cocktail I didn't order: guilt mixed with immense sadness and topped off with fear. Thinking about this unwanted cocktail it was only natural to consider the potent mixed drink forced on my brother. Of course, whatever amount of sadness and pain I felt, it could not compare to the emotions my brother was experiencing. I can only imagine what it feels like to go from being a completely healthy

26 year-old one day, and the next day learn you are going to have to spend an undetermined amount of time battling a life-threatening disease. Considering his emotions and seeing the strength he exhibited throughout his sickness helped me to cope with my feelings.

Throughout my brother's sickness I tried to consider the ways in which I could continue to serve as a source of strength or support to him, as I had been in the past. The most difficult part of this, for me, was living thousands of miles away from him and being weighed down by the burdens of a doctoral program with its never-ending demands. When I saw my brother, during the times he had major surgeries or was receiving chemo, I tried my best to be whatever he told me (or what I sensed) he needed me to be. I tried to tap into our ways of communicating that we always had, as brother and sister. If I thought he needed a laugh and some distraction, I would tell a funny story. If I could tell he needed a rest, I would take my parents out to lunch or go sit with them in the waiting room of the hospital. When he needed someone to run to the grocery store to buy him the fat-free foods he was required to eat following removal of the lymph nodes in this stomach, I came back with bags of items and brainstormed meals for him. When he came home from his second surgery and didn't have to be on a fat-free diet, I baked him several batches of cookies and we watched crappy TV together.

I also realized that there were things I could say to my brother that my parents wouldn't or couldn't. When I first saw him in the hospital I held in my tears for all of about 20 minutes and then I stated the obvious, "it sucks to see you here having to go through this." When I began crying, our parents and my brother cried too, something that they had not yet done together. Our parents tried to be stoic, as positive as possible, and not be angry or upset around him; at that time, however, that approach had trapped the three of them into not sharing their fear and sadness. Afterwards, my parents and brother told me that my acknowledging the elephant in the room and voicing exactly what they had been feeling and had wanted to say (well, maybe not in my exact words), allowed us to come together as a family.

Coping with my brother's sickness was very much a learning process in changing family roles. Although always the big sister, with a desire to protect, I learned that support can be given in many different ways. Sometimes it is batches of cookies and bad television; sometimes it is saying the hard truth and sharing raw emotions. But support also manifests itself in acknowledging the mutuality of need that touches a family when confronted with illness. As much as I've tried to give support to my brother, in truth, he has been my greatest source of strength throughout this process. The way that he confronted and battled his sickness (and continues to do so), and adjusted to all the ups and downs of being ill with grace and courage has solidified for me what I have always known: my brother is a beautiful, amazing person and I am incredibly proud and thankful that I am his sister.

MY COMING OUT AS SICKLY STORY

MANDY EARLEY

I've been chronically ill for at least twelve years, but this last year has been different. Dissatisfied with the useless diagnoses, treatment plans, and prescriptions I'd received from the many doctors I've seen over the years, I decided to take matters into my own hands. And I got better. And better. And then one day I was practically healthy. I was ecstatic, as I finally felt like I was gaining some semblance of control over my life. I wanted so desperately to tell everyone I knew, but quickly realized it wouldn't be so easy. That's because no one really knew that I was sick in the first place.

At first, I just told my closest friends in intimate confidence, and their reactions shocked me. They were completely, unwaveringly supportive, and I learned that many of my friends have similar medical problems, or had been through something similar at some point in their lives... I started telling everyone, and while I can't say their reactions have always been equally affirming, I can say the whole process has been positive and life-changing.

I've realized that talking about sickness is necessary to de-stigmatize illness, communicate limitations, build community between those dealing with chronic illness, learn and disseminate alternative strategies for getting better, and agitate for better health care. It's essential for personal healing and for political change. As a result, this piece is both my personal narrative and a call for my fellow sick folk to come out of the closet.

*   *   *

So where to start? At this point you're probably wondering what's wrong with me. It's a question that sickly people know well. In short, I'm either immunologically fucked or I have too much immunity. I have a whole bunch of auto-immune disorders: asthma, severe seasonal allergies, many food allergies, irritable bowel syndrome, gastro-esophageal reflux disorder (GERD, aka chronic heartburn), eczema, and arthritis. There have been times when I've been on the brink of death, and other (rare) times when I've been "okay" for awhile.

For years I saw a different specialist for each disorder I had. I also had a primary care provider who would document the findings of all of these other doctors, but she could never tell me what it added up to (except for agreeing that I was immunologically fucked). I rode this medical merry-go-round unquestioningly for eleven years, and was sort of satisfied as long as they kept me stocked on my meds and had some sort of scientific explanation for what was wrong with me.

Then last year I hit rock bottom. All of these problems sort of hit at once, but the thing that was really causing me the most trouble was the irritable bowel syndrome. I'd given up most foods other than milk, bread, tomatoes, and meat, but somehow I was still really sick. I already knew I was allergic to all legumes (no more tofu, tempeh, beans, hummus, or veggie burgers) and a lot of vegetables, so I couldn't really handle another food allergy diagnosis. I felt like if they took anything else away from me, I would crack and stab a specialist in the kidney (being sickly, I know just where the kidneys are located).

In any case, I got to a point where my body was hardly digesting food. Almost every meal passed right through me with little thought on the part of my digestive system. It was like there was a knife in my stomach, a fire in my heart, and I was nauseated about half the time. I was also experiencing more headaches, sinus problems, and asthma attacks. I was always run-down and depressed, which is what happens when you're badly malnourished. I felt like I was never going to get better, and was seriously wondering if I had anything left to live for. Somehow I was working my ass off and getting by professionally. God knows how.

I had totally exhausted my options within traditional Western medicine. Every time I saw a specialist they'd rehash the diagnosis of the specialists before them, and it was starting to feel like a waste of my time. I was having a hard time dealing with any asthma triggers at all (household mold, seasonal allergies, exercise, the common cold), and my visits to my asthma doctor were getting increasingly desperate. "So ... if I move to a different kind of house I won't get better... and if I take this medicine I won't get better... and I took that one and I didn't get better... So there's really nothing you can do at all. Nothing that can make me feel alright *ever*..."

The doctor tried to console me by telling me that many people with my disorders live very full lives—with the aid of prescriptions, and by reducing their physical activity, and by not going out too much in the summer (or fall or spring) and by living in the most hypoallergenic accommodations they can find. And, like pulmonary doctors before him, he reminded me that it could be worse. I could have even nastier disorders, or as one specialist once said, "At least it's not lung *cancer*." You're *probably* not going to die. Just be sure not to run or walk too briskly or get a bad cold or eat some soy by accident or get blown over by a strong wind. Given such demotivational diagnoses and treatment plans, I made an appointment to see an acupuncturist because I figured I had nothing to lose. I couldn't feel much worse, could I?

I had no idea just how much a doctor of traditional Chinese medicine could help, and as cheesy as it sounds, Chinese medicine gave me my life back. I have an awesome acupuncturist at Oriental Health Solutions in Durham, NC, and she has actually treated all of my problems successfully. Chinese medicine is a holistic practice, so they look to how certain meta-imbalances affect multiple systems, and as I'd expected, all of these auto-immune disorders ARE related. They believe that the digestive system supports immunity and the lungs, and my acupuncturist said I had to improve my digestion before I could expect to feel better on the asthma and allergies front. I didn't believe it at first, but I figured anything was worth a try at that point.

She put me on herbs to balance my system and digestive enzymes to make up for my pancreatic deficiencies. And much to my surprise *I started digesting food again*. All of a sudden, within a day or so of taking the supplements I was getting nutrition from the things I ate. It wasn't a complete fix, and I'd learn shortly thereafter that my true and worst allergy was milk, but it was a huge improvement. Soon thereafter I gave up milk, and my asthma, allergies, and digestive problems mostly went away.

That's not to say that I'm totally healthy and immunologically fabulous now. I still have to put a lot of work into staying healthy, and staving off my body's natural imbalances. A cold can still be a lot more dangerous for me, and every now and then when I exercise I get that certain "oh, I can't breathe" feeling. I can still be totaled by some milk powder put in bread at a fast food joint or an organic bakery. I'm on a whole anti-inflammatory diet to overcome all of the damage I did to my body by eating allergens for years, and so I generally don't eat sugar, gluten, or yeast in addition to the legumes and dairy I've already given up. It's made it a lot harder to eat out, but I appreciate that it has forced me to eat local, fresh, healthy, and homemade foods. While it's a lot of work, I'm incredibly grateful for the knowledge and treatment options I have, and it's all the better that it came from outside of the traditional medical and food industries.

*   *   *

Initially, the impetus for coming out as sickly came from the changes in my diet. Many of the people in my life couldn't imagine giving up milk, especially since I'd already given up legumes. Between these two restrictions, I can't eat much of what is considered "food" in America today. It's really an alienating experience to walk through a frozen food section or gas station and realize there's almost nothing I can eat. My friends knew that either something was really wrong, or I was just really fucking weird. As great as it is to be weird, I finally started telling people bits and pieces of the story, and eventually the whole story.

I began telling people about how I had undiagnosed digestive problems for all of high school, how the doctors never helped anyway once I was diagnosed, the process by which sickness derailed my graduate education, and how the times when I wasn't returning calls it was often because I was too sick to get out of bed. And I experienced something I didn't expect. I thought it was just a horrible story like any other horrible story, and that they'd hear it, move on, and forget about it. But people's reactions were bigger than that, and it made me realize that chronic illness was bigger than I allowed it to be. It wasn't just a road trip from hell, or a hangover of legendary proportions, or a boring wedding. It really was different than most people's experience of life. Chronic illness had been one of the defining features of my life for years, and somehow I just never told anyone.

This is not to say that talking about my illnesses is always easy or something I want to do all of the time. The single worst thing for me is dealing with other people's lack of understanding of my health problems. It's not surprising that people don't know more about fairly common disorders, given that most of us get our medical knowledge from grade school biology (this is where babies come from + don't do drugs!), but it can get old to be an educator about your illnesses. While you've heard your story a thousand times, and it may be painful, emotionally wrought, or boring to you, it will always be novel, shocking, or fascinating to others. They may ask painful questions about whether you've tried everything you can, whether you have the right diagnosis, how soon you'll get "better," when you think you'll be eating your allergenic foods again, and perhaps worst of all if you may have imagined it or be faking. While these questions are incredibly difficult, and can verge on insensitive, I always keep in mind that these people just don't understand the situation. Illness, or your particular illness, may be completely foreign to a lot of people. The only way they can understand is to discuss the medical condition with them, and often the understanding they gain comes in handy if your limitations are an issue in the future.

The other part I find most difficult to navigate are conflicts with my own radical politics and with the political community to which I belong. While I see my illness and treatment as further evidence that this country's medical and food systems are totally out of control, and have used it to inspire my politics, sometimes people who don't know me think that I'm either not very political or less political because of my limitations. I have to explain to people that I'm still "working up" to cycling, as I still have a hard time biking places with my asthma. I've had to break it to people that I can't eat whatever they found in a dumpster, and it's hard to reveal that my messenger bag is full of supplements, digestive enzymes, asthma inhalers, and epi pens. It was particularly difficult for me as an anti-consumerist to rely on mass-produced products to stay healthy, but luckily with

Chinese medicine I have more natural alternatives. It bothers me that I don't have as much time, flexibility, or energy as some activists I know because I'm already so worn out from taking care of myself, and I feel guilty about not being more involved. Also, I often have to justify my "decision" to work an office job in order to afford healthy, hypoallergenic food, take care of myself, and remain insured. In reality, I feel so grateful that I even have the job that I have, as much as I still dream of a society where health care is not unjustly tied to the ability to work. Many people with chronic illnesses do not have this luxury.

I went through a phase of not telling anyone again just because I was sick of retelling the story, dealing with their disbelief, feeling like I was really different, and worrying about conflicts between sickness and politics. I was feeling better and just wanted to put it away for awhile. But it's still a huge part of my life, something that requires accommodation, and a part of my radical politics, so I couldn't keep from talking about it for long.

So here I am now, telling everyone. As mentioned previously, while the process of coming out as sickly has often been difficult and painful, the moments when people finally get it make it worth it. While I still ask for as few accommodations as possible, being that kind of person, it secretly warms my frosty heart whenever someone says "I made these brownies soy, milk, and gluten free for you." Perhaps more touching are the rare moments where I meet other people that are sickly too, or others with secret food allergies. It is always a moment of triumph, of pleasure in difficulty, when you meet someone who has gone through a similar level of hell. Having the understanding of people who've also worn hospital bracelets is invaluable. It is my hope that by telling my story, and having people tell theirs, we can begin a whole other process of healing. Chronic physical illness has mental, emotional, and social tolls that often take a sideline to whatever is wrong with our tangible bodies, so it's essential to find support, self-respect, and a life worth living, regardless of ability or impairment.

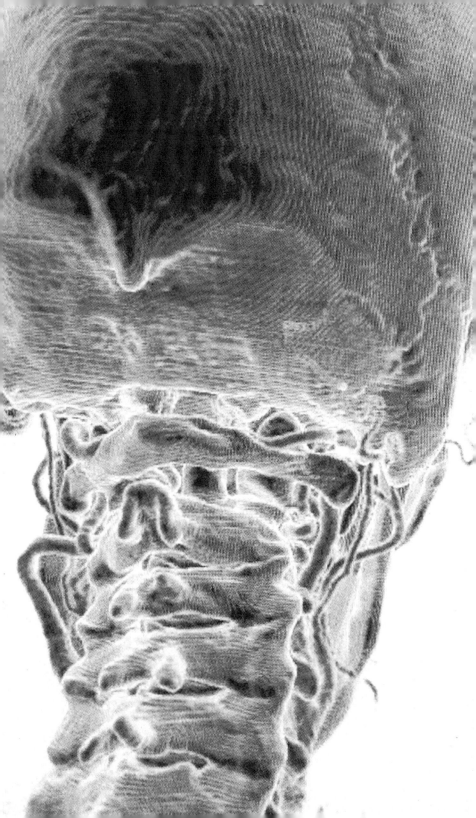

RADICAL HEART SUPPORT

LAUREN DENITZIO

Today I started a month long US tour with my band. We've been together for over four years and have been a large part of what I do and what I'm known for by most of my friends. Recently, I turned 25, quit the job I hated and now make a living doing graphic design and illustration, mostly for bands and record labels. I went to college right out of high school so I could get a "good job" that gave me health insurance and I've worked hard to get to a point where I can live in Brooklyn, go on tour, and not be totally broke. For a lot of people, that isn't all that difficult, but I NEED health insurance, which can be a hard thing to come by. I need health insurance because when I was a kid I was diagnosed with Marfan Syndrome, a connective tissue disorder, which has since affected almost every aspect of my life.

Marfan Syndrome is something that requires regular doctor's visits, but doesn't currently impact my day-to-day life beyond getting out of breath a bit easily and not being able to do heavy lifting. During my adult life, it hasn't been anything I can really complain about, and for that I'm very grateful. My childhood, however, was spent in a back brace, battling severe scoliosis (curvature of the spine) which I had surgically corrected when I was 11.

For most of my life I've also been followed by a cardiologist for a heart condition where my aorta, one of the main valves in your heart, is progressively not doing its job very well. I go see a cardiologist twice a year to make sure I'm not getting worse and am not at a greater risk for an aortic aneurysm than usual. If I were not followed for this, and a developing aneurysm was not caught in time, there is a very good chance I would die. Usually my cardiologist says my condition is just about the same as last time, tells me to call him if I start getting dizzy, and sends me home. But not this time.

Three days ago my cardiologist told me that my heart condition may have gotten a bit worse and I'll need to go back to see him sooner rather than later. My next appointment, in four months, will confirm whether or not I'll need further treatment. And by further treatment I mean have my aorta replaced. I'm not supposed to do anything differently until then, as this may be nothing to worry about, but what a way to start tour.

How do I deal with the fact that I really might have to have heart surgery and have it soon? How did I deal with the fact that I probably can't have children because of this? How did I handle having spinal surgery as a pre-teen? How do I deal with the possibility of a hip replacement or the slight chance I'll lose my eyesight? I'm not totally sure myself. I wish I had an answer for how I get through it, or think about it, if only for my own benefit, let alone that of others.

I do think that one thing that has helped me cope with the uncertainties of my illness is being a part of punk and a radical community. Maybe it's because a lot of us have been through hard times growing up and there's that common bond and understanding. Maybe it's because there's a more open dialogue about support and illness than in other groups. Maybe it's because I can get free therapy out of writing, singing, and playing songs. But whatever it is, having a support system of friends telling me it's okay to be myself and not hide my differences, has given me a better ability to roll with the punches. Being a little "weird" isn't judged harshly, whether it's having blue hair, dressing a little strange or having some pretty cool surgical scars. Needless to say I could've used more of that mentality when I was 5'8" and lanky at age 13.

Dealing with illness and being okay with being "different" has also shaped a lot of who I am as a person. It's why I care more about my friends, working hard at the things I enjoy, and playing music than I do about most material items and monetary wealth. I just have bigger things to worry about. Life is too short to spend it worrying about the latest trend or what other people think of me or the choices I make. So long as I have a roof over my head, I enjoy what I'm doing, and I have health insurance, I'm all set. I'm doing okay right now, but as I have recently found out, that can change in a heartbeat. No pun intended.

Today I get to tour the United States in a van with my friends. Until I go back to see my cardiologist, all I can do is sit back, make sure I take my medication, and enjoy the ride.

555.1

ERICA

Crohn's disease is the shits, literally. Dealing with drastic weight loss, complete lack of energy, months on end of bloody diarrhea, constant pain in the gut, malnutrition, hair loss, not to mention the plethora of side effects that come with all of the medications is never fun. It can be especially damaging to your psyche when you get sick in your teenage years like I did. Right when I was trying to gain independence, I lost control of my own body as well as any control I may have had over how to live my life. Every day and every decision became dictated by my disease and by the rigid regiment of treatments.

However, for some reason, I came to terms with my disease quickly. My condition was diagnosed relatively fast as Crohn's colitis (an autoimmune disease of the large intestine), and I was able to start treatment, so I didn't get far behind in school. I had a supportive network of family and friends, a great doctor, and health insurance through my parents. Crohn's is a chronic disease so it never goes away, although you can treat the symptoms. Sometimes the symptoms will disappear for no good reason at all, and then they will return again, also without warning. As I began college, I had a period of three relatively quiet years. With my disease in relative remission, it seemed like just another routine part of my life. I had to go to the GI doctor occasionally, be comfortable constantly talking about my bowel movements, always know how to get to the nearest bathroom, and get my white blood count tested from time to time.

What I didn't realize in those first few years with the disease was that I had become marked. Despite the fact that I felt like a capable, active, independent person, on paper I was something totally different: uninsurable. Leaving the security of student life (and simultaneously my parent's insurance plan), I have slowly discovered that I am in for a long, hard road.

My first year out of school, I was tipped off that I should not try to get my own health insurance independently. If I tried, I would either get denied or be forced to pay an exorbitant monthly premium. To make matters worse, I was warned that if my coverage was rejected, I would forevermore have to check the box on insurance forms indicating that I had been denied health insurance for medical reasons. Basically, I would be shooting myself in the foot for the rest of my life. So instead, I signed up for a short-term insurance policy, which gave me a year with minimal coverage. It was a crappy plan, but the symptoms of my disease had lessened. I figured I was fine.

Unfortunately, I wasn't fine. Within a few months, my disease returned in full force. With bad insurance, no energy (thus, no job), and no transportation, there was little I could do. I stayed at home, continually getting sicker and sicker. I didn't have the money to pay for the doctors visits, the blood tests, colonoscopies, and Barium drink x-ray procedures needed to investigate the state of my colon. I looked into clinical trials for Crohn's disease since they pay for all of your treatment, but I didn't necessarily trust new drugs. I don't even like to take Tylenol, so an untested treatment was not going to be for me. Instead, I lay in my bed all day, getting up only to go to the bathroom every twenty minutes, most of the time lacking the energy even to sit up. Through all this, I continued to hide the seriousness of the situation from my family and friends. I didn't want them to worry and I wanted to be able to take care of myself.

I finally made a decision that my health was more important than money. I went to the doctor who put me through all the tests and started on a new combination of drugs to get me healthy. This time, however, my flare-ups didn't subside with the drugs, making the next three years a struggle. Juggling medicines, their side effects, Crohn's symptoms, thousands of dollars in medical bills, hours on the phone with the insurance company about EOBs (Explanation of Benefits), not to mention the full-time job I started in order to get insurance (my short-term insurance had run out at this point), I began to realize that this was going to be a lifelong battle. Not just a battle with my disease or a battle to live a relatively "normal" life, but a battle for the ability to pay for treatments and to keep my health insurance coverage.

I don't think there is any person in the United States that hasn't been affected by our country's health insurance policies, either by not having insurance or by having to break her or his back trying to deal with the incomprehensible benefit manuals and customer service representatives. Not to mention that since it is common practice for insurance companies to negotiate a lower bill with doctors' offices, those without insurance are forced to pay higher costs than those who are covered.

With insurance tied to employment, the healthcare industry discriminates against the unemployed, the disabled, undocumented immigrants, the self-employed such as artists and musicians, athletes, part-time workers, and anyone trying not to feed into the system. With preexisting condition clauses, our health insurance system discriminates against anyone with a diagnosis of a severe or chronic illness. With so many procedures needing prior approval, and so many ifs, buts, and ors, the insurance companies are forcing many people to make medical decisions against their better judgment.

Hopefully this system will soon change. However, any system-wide change will take tons of time and compromises, so in the meantime, it is important for those of us with major illnesses to be one step ahead of our insurance companies. I have learned that my health is worth the struggle of dealing with these systems, so that I can lead a full and productive life. However, to the insurance companies, I am still nothing more than my diagnosis, 555.1: Crohn's colitis.

THINGS I AM GRATEFUL I HAD, OTHERWISE I WOULDN'T STILL BE HERE:

- Friends and family that could loan me money to pay medical bills

- Family willing to help keep me up to date about new treatments and clinical trials

- Family and friends that could help me with transportation to the doctor

- No shame about speaking of bloody diarrhea at the dinner table

- Family that provided me a free place to stay when I was too sick to work

- Access to a landline telephone so I could make lengthy calls to the insurance companies in the middle of the day

IMPORTANT THINGS TO KNOW ABOUT HEALTH INSURANCE IF YOU HAVE/HAD A CHRONIC OR SEVERE ILLNESS:

- Be careful applying for your own independent health insurance plan. You may be denied, which can cause greater problems down the line.

- Don't go without insurance for more than 63 days. (You probably shouldn't go without insurance at all, if you can manage it.) 63 is the magic number. If you keep yourself insured with no gaps of more than 63 days, the preexisting condition clause is waived. You will have to get a certificate of credible insurance from your old insurance company though, which usually just takes a phone-in request—or two, or three.

- Your new company might not ask for the certificate of credible insurance, but if you don't send it, they won't cover it, so send it in anyway. Also, keep a copy for yourself so you can send it in again when they claim that they "did not receive it."

- If you are an artist of any sort, consider joining Fractured Atlas, an organization that's sole purpose is providing a group medical insurance plan to artists. It's through Aetna and similar to most other group plans available. Membership to Fractured Atlas does cost something, but it's still much more reasonable than independent insurance. It's not available in all states, so check out their website, www.fracturedatlas.org, to see if it is available where you live. There are also similar programs for other groups/

states, so ask around to see what's out there.

- If you want to check out clinical trials, they usually pay for all your procedures, etc. Check out the NIH's site to search what's being tested. (http://clinicaltrials.gov) HOWEVER, ONLY DO TRIALS THAT ARE IN PHASE 3 OR 4. In those phases they know the side effects and are usually honing in on the proper dosages, i.e., they are fairly sure it won't accidentally kill you.

- Get in touch with a foundation focusing on your illness. The people there may be able to help find you money to pay for expensive treatments.

- Talk with the social worker at your hospital. They can help connect you with resources.

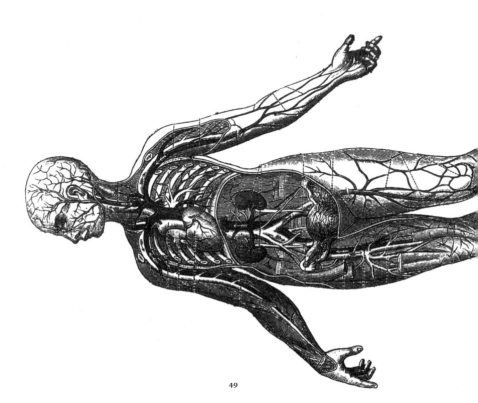

CUT ACROSS THE DOTTED LINE

TESSA PETROCCO

Around one in the afternoon, the chalky aftertaste of codeine erupts in my mouth…except there's no pill in sight. My body still craves it fifteen years later.

Every downpour is a reminder of my past. "It's just the aches that come along with getting older, Tessa," my parents said.

"I've been old since I was eight years old," I respond.

Silence.

*   *   *

Most kids who are eight years old are learning their times tables, having their first slumber parties and playing flashlight tag until late hours of the night. I wasn't like most kids.

I started out just like them. I joined a soccer team, which quickly became my entire reason for being. I had an entire neighborhood of friends and even had boys who liked me.

Then it happened.

During a particularly exciting soccer game the summer going into third grade, we were tied with the undefeated team. I had the ball at my feet, quickly approaching the goal, when all of a sudden I felt a pop. I fell to my knees in agony. I don't think I stopped crying until my parents rolled me out of the hospital after my surgery a few days before Christmas.

I was diagnosed with a rare degenerative disease known as Legg-Calvé-Perthes where the hip joint suffers a loss of bone mass that leads to the collapse of the joint itself. In my case, the femoral artery in my hip had stopped delivering blood to the ball of my femur and caused it to shatter.

I was given two options: to operate on the hip joint, which would entail reconstructing the hip, placing it for 8-to-10 months using metal rods and later on removing said rods, or to wear a semi-permanent leg brace for two years.

The leg brace meant transferring to a school for kids with special needs, and I didn't want that, so I told them to cut me open.

I told my mom I wanted her there with me in the operating room, should anything happen to me. Even at such a young age, I knew there were always complications with surgeries, and tearfully, she agreed.

As I was going under anesthesia, my mom's hand in one of my hands and a white, stuffed cat, named Harley after my real cat, in the other, I suddenly became fearful of what was going to happen. The coming months hit me all at once and the fact I was medically delirious didn't help matters. For all I knew, my last moments on Earth would be filled with fearful tears. I clutched onto my mom's hand for dear life and as I passed out, prayed she'd be there when I woke up. *If* I woke up.

But I did wake up, and she was there alongside my dad. At that moment, I knew what unconditional love truly felt like and it hasn't left since.

Like most people who go through massive reconstructive surgery, I gained weight. It's human nature to have it get to you after a while, feeling hopeless and helpless, but when you have hundreds of students reminding you on a daily basis on just how big you've gotten by means of names like "Tessa Monster" or "Pink Flamingo," it's harder than most. I tried to remain strong and not let it get to me, though.

Several months after my second surgery, this time to take the metal pins out of my hip, I had begun growing. I was excited. Growing meant I was normal again.

*   *   *

By the time I reached thirteen, I was 5-feet, 6-inches, had more curves than most 13 year old girls should and started dealing with typical body issues. The fact that I had a 9-inch scar on my hip with another 3-inch one above it stopped me from showing any sort of skin, especially in the summer. As far as I was concerned, bathing suits were an abomination.

That year brought on another sore subject for me...literally. The leg in which I had surgery on was starting to pose a new problem: back pain. Because the leg's growth is stunted during the healing process and my body continued to grow anyway, I had a leg shortening of about $\frac{1}{2}$-inch difference in my right leg (my surgery leg).

I tried orthopedic shoes at first, but the kids at school were relentless. They made me feel like a bigger freak than I already felt I was (although I'm sure the baggy, weird clothes and dark makeup didn't help either). Finally, I decided to go with a discreet, small insole lift that went inside my shoe, the closest thing I could have to just wearing shoes normally.

Sometimes I joked about it. Sometimes I *had* to joke about it. I'd call myself

Granny or Gimp on a weekly basis. My friends called it my "pimp walk." I'd even contemplated getting a tattoo when I turned eighteen that said, "Limpin' ain't easy," in hopes to make it easier to deal with.

Every morning when I put my shoes on, however, I'd see it and it would remind me it's not easy to deal with.

* * *

Within the next couple years, I had seen my orthopedic doctor a handful of times with concerns about my joint pain.

The first appointment, shortly after I turned eighteen, started out routine. Essentially, since he's a pediatric orthopedist, I had one last hurrah appointment, giving me the clear to lead a normal life.

However, things quickly went from "normal checkup" to "here's how your life is going to pan out." He told me that unlike the other patients in his case study, I was one of few who didn't heal as desired. My hip joint was permanently misshapen which would cause pain throughout my life more so than his other Legg-Calvé-Perthes cases. Regardless of what I did, I would need a hip replacement by mid-life.

To be entirely honest, I saw that coming. What I didn't see coming was that he said any sort of job I wanted to do involving being on my feet would be out of the question unless I wanted to bump my replacement surgery up 10-20 years.

I wanted to be a filmmaker. So, instead of being on my feet and behind the camera like I had originally planned, I took a different route and studied to be a screenwriter or video editor instead. That way, I could do what I wanted and extend the life of my natural hip.

Of course, I hadn't been that calm at first. No one ever takes bad news lightly. I thought it was the end of my reason for being at that point. But, as life goes, you learn to adapt and figure out ways to do what you need and/or want to do.

With a massive weight gain and increase of joint pain under my belt, at age twenty I went to see Georgie (the nickname I gave my doctor as a kid) again.

This time, I was a little more rocked. Now standing at 5-feet, 9-inches (or 5-feet, 8 ½-inches depending on which leg I'm standing on) and weighing 265 pounds, he told me that if I didn't drop weight, I'd need a hip replacement by 30. Essentially, since my hip joint is two times as sensitive as a normal hip, with every step I take, two times my weight is stressed on my hip. That was over 400 pounds of pressure on my hip several hundred times a day. I was really starting to understand just how serious this disease was years after being "cured."

I dropped 85 pounds within the next year.

*   *   *

Now, at twenty-three, I wish I could say, "Oh, I dropped all this weight and I feel amazing and life is perfect!" That's not true, of course. With every disease and every illness comes struggle, even years after the initial symptoms have been treated. There's a reason why remission exists.

I could have chosen to let the disease take me over. I could have taken a job that would later cost me months of surgery and physical therapy. I could have become an automated medication machine, thinking the future of my pain lies within a pill. I could have stayed at 265 and had the replacement done by 30, but chances were I'd gain even more weight after the surgery and end up bed-ridden by middle age.

Life, as I knew it, could have ceased to exist.

So, instead of letting the disease beat me, I've decided to beat it. It's a day-by-day process and some days are naturally better than others. I still ache when it rains, I still get pops and cracks (especially when going up stairs), I still have days where looking at my scar in the mirror causes more pain than the joint itself, but in the end...I'm living life how I want to.

This is my one shot, and it lies in my hands...or in my case, my hip.

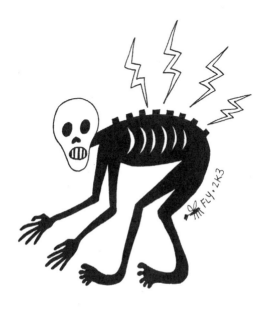

CLEARING HEAD: A STORY ABOUT MIGRAINES

BRITTANY SHOOT

How I have long conceptualized my migraines has perhaps the greatest impact on how I experience them.

For some, migraines are visual impairments, temporary blindness, and nausea. For others, the pain – either in your temples, across your forehead, or down your neck and shoulders – makes you twist into strange positions, the oddest pressure points acting as temporary relief. Some people avoid certain trigger foods and alcohol. Some disappear for days at a time into dark, cold, quiet rooms, the only respite from the hellish onslaught of a variety of symptoms and effects.

Speaking from a perspective of Western medicine, migraines can be caused by neurological disorders, head or spinal cord trauma, the strain of undiagnosed poor eyesight. Various persuasions of Eastern medicine will blame the pain on internalized stress, bodily imbalances, a build-up of toxins, misaligned qi, and the obvious bad sleep and diet. In my experience, migraines are often the result of causes from both philosophies.

Migraines are an isolating condition because of the literal solitude that can be required for healing. In my case, a cold, dark, quiet room is usually necessary, which means you not only get to enter a potentially boring, lonely space for an indefinite amount of time; others around you are also forced to be quiet and live/work in dimly lit spaces. You also have no idea when the pain might end. Your medication might not work. You might not have medication. It could be another day before this subsides. You have to start canceling things. I usually end up apologizing to several people.

My battle with migraines began when I was around eight years old. My family life was less than ideal, with a stepmother who regularly berated me behind my disbelieving father's back and a mother who wasn't convinced such a young child could get such ferocious headaches. Few people in my family believed in my soon-to-be chronic condition, and from the beginning, this established an atmosphere of guilt, shame, and quick fixes to feel better again as soon as possible with no emphasis on the root causes, what could make stress manifest in such a difficult way for a sensitive pre-pubescent girl.

Two main things seem to complicate the illness the most: that it is mostly an invisible condition, not easily seen and identified by others; and that while many people experience a wide range of difficult headaches and occasional nausea, most people are not rendered helpless for days at a time due to either symptom. For many, a migraine is a disease of convenience, an excuse to demand meals at a certain time, to generally act finicky in public, or alternately, to stay home and sleep.

In activist circles, I have taken my share of criticism for most commonly failing to show up somewhere because I'm sick – ashamed I am not present and therefore not always forthcoming about my absence, knowing the reactions I face – or for not acting in ways other people find healthy, though they have little idea what health means to me.

"Gee, you take a lot of medication, don't you?" Even on paper, this statement sounds full of blame, not concern. "What did you eat?" "Have you had enough to drink?" While these may be statements of worry from people who like to problem-solve, they inevitably force a sick person to explain him/herself. As most sensitive people with chronic conditions will tell you, we know every trigger by now. We know how to handle these things. The lack of trust others put in us when they question our ability to care for ourselves is confusing, irritating, sad, humiliating, and disempowering. It can prompt defensive responses and anger. It may immediately make a sick person worse, particularly if their condition is stress-related.

As long as my migraines have been misunderstood, I've also misunderstood the magnitude of my problem. Feeling guilty, I would attempt to quash sickness with pills and a cold cloth, enough to still go to a meeting, to work. In forcing myself into wellness that was a lie, I've ended up puking in rental cars, on the side of the road, leaning out of stopped taxis, whose drivers are patient enough to wait for me and hand me a tissue; in someone's front yard, in my own front yard, in public garbage cans, in an amusement park, in an alley in Dublin on a vacation. The collective humiliation of these events only reinforced that it was my fault. I was sick, and then I made it worse.

Only through allied friendships, with those who also experience chronic conditions or who can empathize with my guilt-ridden pain, did I find enough space to accept that I needed larger scale healing, to stop blaming myself, to start learning that my anger towards others' misunderstanding was not a solution. And while I don't yet know how to combat the negativity of others, I do know what I need.

I need for people to sit with me, to touch me gently, to love me. Often, my partner takes this role, fetching medication and holding my hand, saying, "I'm sorry you feel so badly." My best friend has literally held my hair back, then gently put me to bed. Even when I was young, I could count on one person, my empathetic stepfather, to run to the store for 7-Up, to come into my dark room and rub my head and shoulders. Validation in a time of remorseful sickness is truly restorative. To feel less alone is deeply comforting, as is the knowledge you can allow another to care for you when you simply cannot care for yourself.

I also need to be able to out myself to others, particularly activists who sometimes seem to only have one goal. I want to build community where I can be honest about my sickness, as well as my fears. I want that community to include working on larger causes while accepting everyone's limitations. When I join a group, make a new ally or friend, I need to be able to say, "Sometimes I will get sick" without being treated like an exaggerating, unenthusiastic nuisance. I believe owning my illness, without justifying it, is the first step. The next one begins with everyone else.

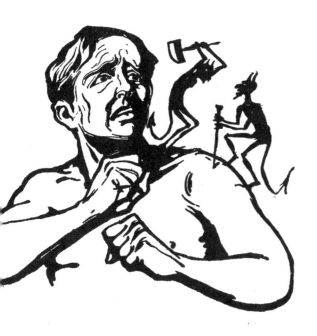

WHAT I'VE LEARNED FROM CHRONIC LYME DISEASE

ANDREA RUNYAN

I've had Lyme disease for seven months. The persistent fatigue and pain, not to mention the cognitive and emotional dysfunction, have made Lyme probably the hardest thing I've ever experienced. However, it's exactly these challenges that have taught me some important life lessons.

I've learned:

1) DON'T WORRY ABOUT ACCOMPLISHING A LOT.

I used to care a lot about using my time well and accomplishing as much as possible. I was one of those people who answered "how was your day?" with "great, I got a lot done," or "bad, I didn't get anything done."

However, Lyme disease put me into a time dilation where not only does it take longer to do things, but now I need to rest and sleep more.

Needless to say, I learned to reduce my demands on myself. I came to see that as long as I take care of the important things, it's not so terrible if I don't get much done in a given day. I slowly escaped the paradigm in which the purpose of each day - and of one's life - is to accomplish as much as possible. I'm coming to see that there's enough time in life and that life is not necessarily characterized by scarcity.

2) PAMPER YOURSELF.

Before getting Lyme disease, I got by without doing much for myself at all. I probably thought I did things for myself, but they were useful things that were more for my benefit than my enjoyment.

But once saddled with the pain and mental confusion of Lyme disease, I needed something strong to counteract the badness of my life and to keep my mind distracted and out of its strange Lyme patterns. I needed to do things that reliably boosted my happiness and gave me something to look forward to.

I watched the TV series The Office on DVD, read the Dykes to Watch Out For comic books (since I couldn't concentrate enough to read regular books), ate yummy food, took bubble baths, and colored in coloring books. I learned to do things FOR myself, not just to demand things FROM myself.

3) THINK ABOUT THINGS HOW YOU WANT TO THINK ABOUT THEM.

According to the usual paradigm, Lyme disease has been a terrible thing for me. I haven't been able to do much for half a year, many of my organs are now damaged with toxins, and most painfully, people who are close to me judge me because they don't understand what I'm going through.

But from my own perspective, Lyme disease been a wonderful learning opportunity, like a challenging graduate program that demands sustained effort, creative thinking and troubleshooting. My assignments are not written homework, but rather crises to survive, bacteria to eliminate, and symptoms to alleviate. Though I won't get any letters after my name, "graduating" from Lyme disease will be something of which I am as proud of as any degree.

4) DON'T WORRY WHAT OTHER PEOPLE THINK ABOUT YOU/TRUST YOURSELF. THEY'LL NEVER KNOW THE WHOLE SITUATION, SINCE YOU'RE THE ONLY ONE WHO EXPERIENCES YOUR BODY AND MIND.

Lyme disease and its coinfections strongly affect the nervous system and can impair memory, concentration, and emotional control. To the person experiencing these symptoms, it might be obvious that the symptoms are due to Lyme disease, but an outside observer might not realize that infections can cause such extreme psychiatric symptoms. In my case, I encountered many situations in which I could tell Lyme disease was affecting me, but an outside observer might have thought I was having separate psychiatric problems.

For example, one time when I stopped my antibiotics, I developed such an altered response to stress that I broke down, shaking and crying, in my doctor's office. Not being Lyme-literate, she suggested that I might have an anxiety disorder, but I knew from what I had read about Lyme and from how strange my body felt that I was experiencing Lyme disease symptoms, not a separate psychiatric condition. It was hard being told that my problems were in my head, but experience taught me to trust my own experiences and not to care if other people thought I had a mental condition.

As another example, I haven't been able to work yet since getting Lyme. Sometimes people wonder why I can't work, since I look well enough, but they can't see the chronic pain, the excessive sleep need, the difficulty standing in place for more than a few seconds, and the low stress tolerance that I experience. Thus, I've learned not to care if people think that I'm malingering, since I can tell that, in fact, I'm working hard to get better.

I'm coming to see that even in non-Lyme-related cases, other people probably don't understand where I'm coming from, since they don't experience my body, emotions, or history. In general, I don't need to worry if people think badly of me without understanding the whole situation.

All in all, Lyme disease has probably been the hardest single experience of my life, but that's what's made it so growth-promoting for me. I hope that our culture will see chronic illness not as a sign that person is lazy, self-indulgent, or undesirable but as an indication that they've had the occasion to learn many important lessons.

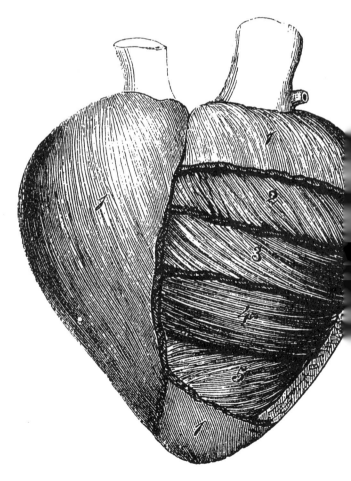

The following is an excerpt from

MY BODY IS THE BRILLIANT CONTRADICTION: FIVE MEDITATIONS ON BEING ILL

KRISTIN ALYSIA PAPE

ONE: IN WHICH I DECIDE TO WRITE PUBLICLY ABOUT BEING ILL

MS, like cancer, turns the body on itself. It stirs a war there; it makes divisions, a Gordian knot of negative spaces. In the gaps are always little murders: cells, stabilities. The first time I saw MRI photographs of my brain, dotted with the milky little galaxies of lesions, the impossibly thin line of my skull circling it like a child's chalk drawing, fragile as sparrow legs, the first time I saw that, the world swung up under me and I went down. Disease is a brilliant contradiction. The foreign body's mine.

Living with disease does this: without your willing it, the secret parts of you light up and burn too intimate and familiar.

After the iced lick of alcohol swab, you press needle through skin, down through the pop and grit of muscle. Push the plunger slow and know that what makes the cold burn near the bone is foreign, is poison, is not really your choice at all. Count hours until what always comes next finally comes: nausea, weariness, grinding aches in your bones so keen you're paralyzed for long minutes. Know that for a day, your lungs won't give you enough air. You'll smell unfamiliar: sweet musk of your skin replaced by the sharp hospital smell of disinfectant. Think of stopping the treatment that only makes you sick so that you don't get sicker. Dream, guilty, of release: wheelchair, numbness, the body finally silenced, nothing left to be done. Tell yourself you're just tired. Irrational. Know you'll dutifully do it, the shot, again, on schedule.

Disease is a foreign brilliance; my body is the contradiction.

Aphasia: sometimes the word I want goes dancing off without me, as weightless and flirtatious as a wind-born seed spore, a papery butterfly I can't catch, leaving me the wrong one, leaving me a foreign tongue, a world of solid, nameless things. Elevator goes often. Often, *umbrella*. *Escalator*. *Plate*. My lover asks, when I'm stammering after *blessing* or *hairbrush*, "Is it the M.S.?" A momentary wince of pain, a lapse of memory one afternoon, sets suspicion in: I imagine the bloom and seep of new lesions like ink spots. Like feathery chrysanthemums opening, a spray of fireworks, the gamma ray bursts of collapsing stars.

Friends say, "You look so very good, you don't look sick, you must be getting better." It's less description than demand.

My body's a lesson, a warning, a needle, a foreign tongue, a seed spore I can't catch. My body's a nameless, disobedient thing. Call it *elevator, umbrella, lesion* or *sparrowleg*. Call it *inkspot*. *Chrysanthemum*. *Blessing*.

TWO: IN WHICH I SEARCH FOR A TRANSLATION

In English, we have no language for pain. We speak only in metaphors, indirect and unsatisfying, never quite up to the task. Our metaphors for pain are always about violence to the body (to paraphrase Elaine Scarry), as if to conjure up the image of the harm will accurately account for the pain that results: *I feel a searing pain in my arm. I have a pounding headache. The news of her death was gut-wrenching.* I'm trying to find a more accurate language, one that accounts for the pain of disease without casting disease as a violent opposition, an enemy army. Being constantly at war is exhausting. Disease has become the murderer and mother, my faithless but familiar lover. I've made my home there, uneasily, tenuously, like a squatter finds home in darkened, empty buildings.

Some days I forget I'm sick. When the morning's brilliantly sunny and cool and I wake up early and not tired, when my body feels good because I don't feel it at all, I can live a sweet and temporary fiction. I could be anybody, and I could strike out, a rudderless little ship, with nothing at all in my pockets, hip soundtrack swinging in my head, or slide shipless into the day, no fear of drowning.

Most days, this is impossible. Though they say it's unhealthy, I can't help thinking of myself as a sick person. Even the days when my body cooperates, when the MS seems to be hibernating, there's the diabetes, which means knowing the exact level of sugar in my blood, controlling my chemistry with juice and insulin, paying keen attention to each stutter, shake or hunger pang that may mean danger approaching. It means always carrying a blood test kit, identification, packs of juice, emergency money. It means never having empty hands. I'm connected to a machine—an insulin pump—every minute of my life. It looks like a beeper, except that it's attached to me by a tube I insert under the skin of my stomach. I can take it off temporarily, for a shower or for a little rest, but for an hour at most, which I stretch willfully like a child stretches the hour before bedtime. When I eat, I must press buttons to tell the pump to deliver more insulin to my body. I must remember to change my battery, change my insulin, change the needle, check for air bubbles in the tube. The skin of my stomach is pocked red with welts, the scars of previous tubes. They take months to heal and disappear; I'm always making new ones. I keep the pump hidden in the waistband of my pants. When I'm hot, it presses sweat to my skin; when I toss in my sleep, the tube tangles around my waist, umbilical, and I dream I'm caught by something dangerous in the cold water dark.

It's a constant reminder of what I'm moored to. It's a constant reminder of what's missing in me, the dead spaces my body makes with its cellular suicides.

The pain I've got no language for isn't the body pain of needles or bones. For that, there's metaphor: *burn grind sting wince. Blood and bruise.* The pain I've got no language for is slow and warm and sweet as lake water, familiar and constant as my own breath. Pain is the pure unspeakable language; my body's untranslatable, dumb.

What kind of numbness is it? My neurologist is well-meaning, but it's been more than a year since my right hand's come undone. The stunned nerves always vibrate, as if I've banged my funny bone, or fallen asleep on my arm. It's a speechless hand; it feels thick, full of pins, clumsy and foreign. Buttons bedevil me, my handwriting's a messy child's scrawl. By some cosmic joke, it can still feel burn, cut, sting, but not a silk skirt, not the stroke of skin. What do you call that kind of numb?

I call it sorrow, anger, fatigue. When I stumble to keep up with friends in the street, when I hide inside on sunny days because the heat makes my body senseless, when insulin reactions come three in a row to send me shaking, nauseated, weak-legged down, I name it grief, dread, loneliness. I name it humiliation.

When we lie curled together in the sea-dark, my lover traces gooseflesh along my clavicle, her bare-legged beauty glowing like milkweed in the half-light. She tugs at the little tube that snakes between us and she whispers: *Why don't you take it off now and be a real live girl for a while?*

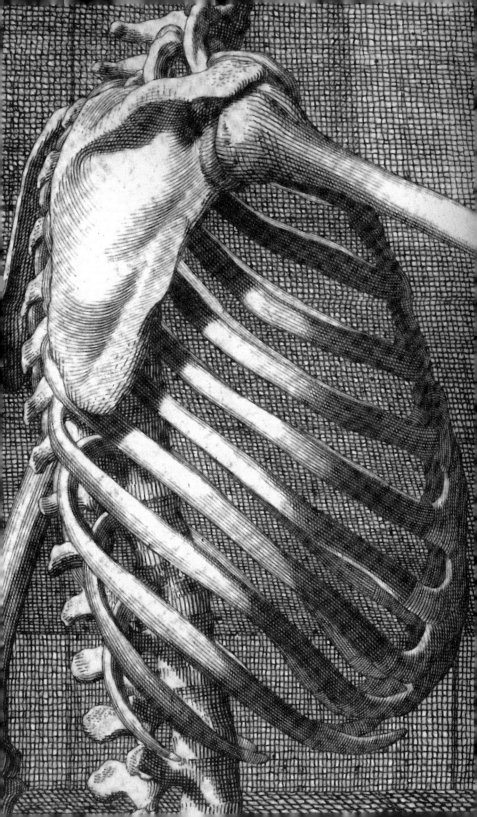

ILLNESS AND SUPPORT

BEN HOLTZMAN

Eighteen months ago—at the age of twenty six—I was diagnosed with cancer. Since that time, I've had three major operations and several months of chemotherapy. I have also experienced numerous other, perhaps less obvious, effects of having a serious, sustained physical health problem: navigating through a purposely disempowering world of doctors, treatments, and hospitals; being truly faced with my own mortality for the first time; losing control of my body; reorienting how I thought I was going to be able to live my life; having the constant threat of complete financial instability; and feeling more scared, confused, and vulnerable than I ever thought possible.

Throughout this time, I've been on the receiving end of a wealth of support from family and friends; this support has made it possible to live through this experience instead of being overcome by it. However, I've also experienced numerous instances in which friends—including many within punk/DIY/activist scenes— have not known how to respond and, in some cases, have not responded at all. Upon diagnosis and a later recurrence, friends I knew for over a decade were barely able to say more than a few words to me; others who I had more recently become close to suddenly drifted away.

In talking to many other people struggling with illness and disease, I've found that the experience of having a health crisis compounded by a lack of support, if not abandonment, is not uncommon. This can be more terrifying than the illness itself.

It's important that those of us within radical/DIY scenes address how we can better support ourselves and our loved ones as well as how we can reconstruct our communities to better address issues of care and support. This article is meant to initiate a dialogue on the issue of support and physical illness by addressing some practical aspects of what may work well and less well in providing support to someone with a serious, sustained physical health problem (in particular, this article focuses on when that person is someone you would consider a friend). Of course, every diagnosis is different and, more importantly, every individual is different. While differences in diagnosis, prognosis, age, gender, insurance, culture, financial status, spirituality, personality and your particular relationship to the person will necessitate different approaches and types of support, what follows is intended to be a useful starting point.

I want to acknowledge that I have felt conflicted about writing an article on support, because I immediately thought to times that I have come up short in this area, not just around issues of illness, but also around the many other situations when support is crucial: friends who have lost loved ones, friends who have had to support members of their immediate family through illness, people in radical circles who have gone to prison. I think of all the times I've made mistakes in how I handled a situation or withdrawn or could have said something different or better. While working on this article, I've come to realize how getting better at support is a process (and not necessarily a linear one). These situations bring us face to face with our own fears and with the most unpleasant aspects of life, even when we are not the ones directly experiencing them. We face a great challenge when we are bold enough to attempt to engage with and improve on how we respond.

This is certainly true for illness. Illness is considered a private topic. We may not have needed to give any thought to illness and support until we've learned that one of our friends—or ourselves—has been diagnosed. Most of us haven't been raised with an understanding of the complexities of how to respond to a situation such as a friend being diagnosed with a serious illness or disease. I think it's important to acknowledge and appreciate this, and understand that you are in no way a "bad" person if you do not immediately know how to respond and provide support to someone dealing with illness. However, if someone that you care about is impacted by illness, it is important not to be complacent in this position and, if you are able, to try to take the initiative to help provide support.

This can start in simple and seemingly insignificant ways. People who initially find out that a friend has been diagnosed with a serious health issue often say that their mind goes blank when they try to think of what to say and that they fear saying the wrong thing. This often results in the person not saying anything. This, in most cases, is the biggest mistake someone can make: people with illness most often want to talk about it and almost everyone at least wants it acknowledged. Saying something—even something small—is almost always better than not saying anything at all. Most people struggling with illness I've talked to have painful memories of certain friends or community members who never even said any words of support to them or who drifted away from them completely after their diagnosis.

If your mind goes blank, remember what you know about this person. You probably know a lot. That's why she or he is a friend. It can be very helpful to use what you know about your friend as a starting point to think about how they might want you to react and what might be helpful to them. It may also be useful to recall a time that you were most scared and frightened to empathize with what your friend is going through and to think about what was helpful and not helpful to you at that time (remembering, of course, that every situation is different, particularly if your experience did not deal with a health crisis). If you still do not know what to say, then acknowledging this and expressing your desire to nonetheless support the person will likely still mean a lot, e.g. "I do not know exactly what to say at this time, but I did want to at least let you know that I am here for you..."

While it is important to say *something* to your friend, it does of course matter what you say and what you do. If you feel that you can provide more than just words of encouragement, the following are suggestions about what people often find helpful and less helpful in being supported.

Numerous books have been written on caregiving and all of them essentially boil down to the following guiding principle in providing support: *learn to listen*. Keep your ears and eyes open and listen to what your friend says. Your friend will most often serve as your guide in helping you to better support her, so long as you actively listen. Listen without judgment, interrupting, or feeling like you have to provide an answer or solution. Also, if you still do not know what the person wants or needs, do not be afraid to ask, instead of assuming.

You may find it useful to read about your friend's diagnosis and condition. If you have a better understanding of what the diagnosis means and what the person will need to go through, you will likely be better informed about how you can support them through it. However, it's important to keep in mind that you should always ask permission before informing your friend about any news or new studies and that you should not give unsolicited advice unless it is welcomed by your friend. People dealing with illness are generally flooded with information and juggling various potential treatment decisions. Adding more information or advice without permission can just make the experience additionally overwhelming.

Similarly, if you knew someone who had the same issue as what your friend has been diagnosed with, it may be tempting to use this knowledge to try to provide some insight. This may be helpful, but remember that an experience with one person does not make you an expert in the condition and that every person experiences a diagnosis differently (both physically and mentally). Be careful not to assume that you automatically know what your friend is going through. Also, never share horror stories about someone you know who has had the same or similar disease.

Another thing that people experiencing sickness often find less than helpful is the 'non-specific offer' of help: "Let me know if there's anything I can do." This is certainly a warm sentiment, but it in some ways passes the buck: you've made the offer and now it's the onus of the person who is sick to come back to you. This can assume that the person dealing with sickness is going to ask for help. It is often very difficult to do this. Someone's lack of asking may not necessarily mean that there is a lack of need. Your friend may find it more helpful if you spend a little bit of time thinking about what the person might really need and then specifically ask about that task. For example: would it be helpful if I accompanied you to the doctor? Would you like me to help you research treatment options? I'd like to do your laundry, would that be something you would want? If you are worried about your medical bills, would you like me to brainstorm ideas for alleviating the financial burden? Do you need help taking care of your pets? Can I take you out to lunch or make/bring you a meal for dinner? If your friend does not need something this week, it does not mean that he won't need something next week. Check in again (and then again).

It can also be important to allow your friend to voice frustration or anger and to avoid trying to put a positive spin on something. Anger and frustration are perfectly valid responses, at least some of the time, to dealing with a serious diagnosis that is unfair, unwanted, undeserved, and utterly life-changing. No person who is sick should be made to feel that they have to be positive all the time. If someone is able to maintain a positive attitude and outlook most of the time, they still have a right to feel negative at other times. Instead of invalidating your friend's feelings or telling your friend how to feel, try to actively understand and acknowledge their feelings.

While I think the fear of "saying the wrong thing" is overstated, there are a number of phrases that can often be less than helpful. One is "everything is going to be just fine." While it can be important to be positive and assuring to your friend, these types of statements can come off as downplaying a serious situation that your friend is going through. Similarly, saying "it could be worse" is making a judgment that only the person with illness has the right to determine for themselves. Also, "you should..." or "you've got to..." are typically not statements that are going to help your friend, at least if phrased in that manner. Finally, when a friend of mine with a very serious diagnosis was told "you've gotten this because you can handle it," it was the closest she came in her life to spitting in someone's face!

An illness also often means that the context and way you enjoy your friend's company may need to shift. What your friend can do physically at times (or possibly all the time) may be limited. One important way to support someone is by continuing to include them in social plans and to work around their restrictions. For example, if your friend has just had surgery and can't leave her apartment, offer to bring over a few movies and hang out. If the illness or being on particular medication means that he can't drink, suggest plans that do not involve bars and/or partying. If your friend is struggling with a digestive disorder and having a flare up during which eating out is hard, offer to make dinner following the guidelines for what she can eat. For someone with illness, it's very easy to begin to feel like a burden to your friends when you're sick. Reorienting social plans around your friend's needs so that they continue to be able to hang out can be tremendously important.

However, it is also important to be mindful of how someone who is sick may not feel like hanging out or even calling back. When I was in chemotherapy, I was too exhausted to see people and felt too miserable to continually have phone conversations in which I told people how terrible I felt. These conversations generally didn't make me feel any better, so after the first round of treatment, I decided that I needed to have brief periods of being out of contact during each subsequent round of chemotherapy. Some of the best messages I received during these times were ones in which friends just called or sent a nice handwritten note to say that they were thinking about me. I knew that they were not expecting a call back if I was not up for talking but that they would talk all night if I was. Calls that were much less helpful were ones in which people guilted me in to calling back so that they could be assured everything was okay or ones in which people asked for the latest update for what was going on as if they had simply wanted to do their job of 'checking in.'

For friends who are dealing with chronic problems (or recurrences), it's also important not to assume that things will always get easier over time. While the time after diagnosis is often the hardest, people who continually have to deal with their illness may find it difficult to keep up their stamina and optimism. It is not uncommon to hear people dealing with illness speak of the support they received being greatest after their diagnosis but then dwindling as time passed, even though they still needed understanding if not outright care from those around them. Multiple stages of disease, new attempts to try different forms of medicines/procedures, and/or successes and setbacks in treatment may bring additional life changes to your friend and may mean continual shifts in how you can best support your friend. Life may never return to status quo. Even if your friend isn't dealing with a chronic problem, be aware of how changes to circumstances or things like check-up appointments or anniversaries of diagnosis can stir up a lot of emotion and make these particular times more difficult.

Two final bits of advice: do not underestimate the importance of reminding someone how much you love and care for them and how you are there to support them. Also, remember the importance of touch: holding someone's hand or giving them a hug (if that's appropriate and welcome) seems insignificant, but can make a huge difference.

I hope that this article helps to further a dialogue about support and illness, particularly within radical/DIY/punk scenes. There is so much more that can be said about what I've written here; this article could easily be expanded into an entire book. I hope that others will add to this topic and also address the many related issues in future articles. As I noted, most likely nothing I've written can be applied to everyone at all times and support will need to be applied in different ways based on the person (this is one of the many reasons why communication and listening to your friend are so critical!) Getting better at providing support is a process and one that with effort each of us can improve on to better help our friends and move us towards reconstructing our communities around provisions of care.

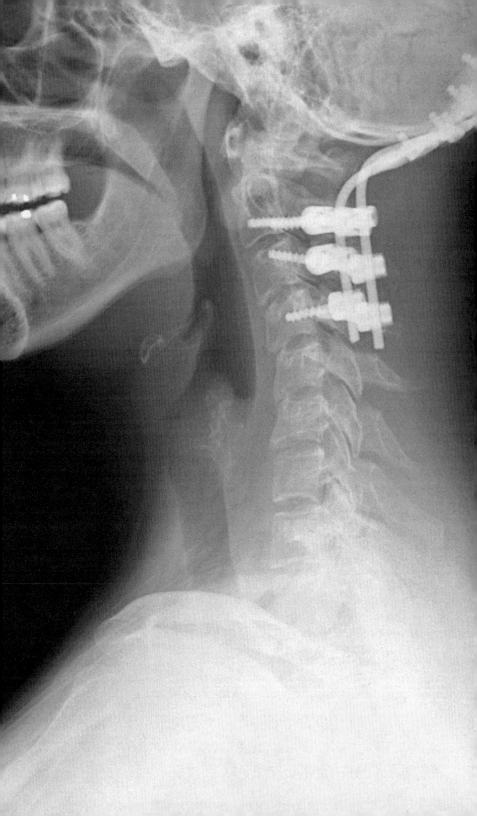

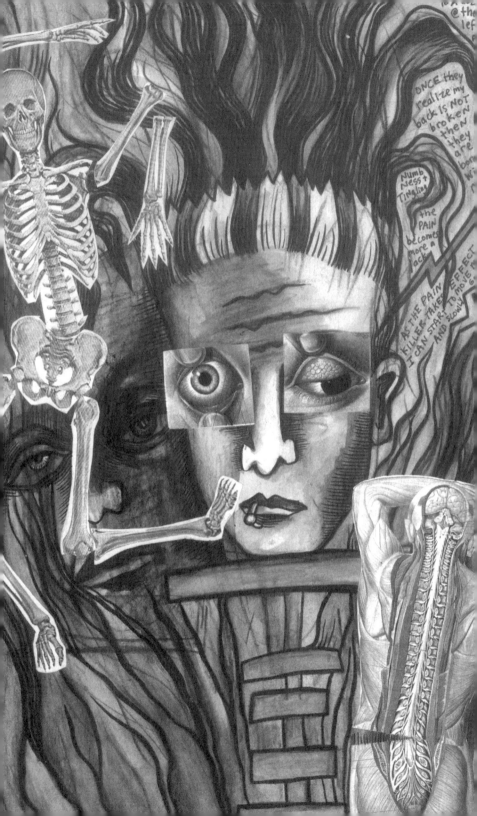

THE OTHER SIDE OF SUPPORT

EMA

Since being diagnosed with a Mulitple Sclerosis (MS) (a chronic autoimmune disease that affects the central nervous system) two years ago, I have gone through and continue to go through a series of findings: finding out about my body, my illness, my strengths and limitations and my shifts in perspective. But because nothing is ever only about me or you – and it is always about us and we – the last two years have also been a time of discovery when it comes to seeking support and being a supportee. In my previous life, I didn't have much experience in seeking and managing support as I'm an independent person who enjoys keeping certain aspects of my life to myself. But one of the first things I did was tell my parents, partner and close friends. It was intrinsic … and necessary for more than emotional reasons.

We all need and desire support. But even if it is a natural thing, it can feel difficult to find and awkward to maneuver. There are plenty of tips and guidelines for the supporters, but this piece is for the supportees (these roles are fluid and ever shifting, so it may help to be familiar with both!). The following are guidelines I have gathered from my individual experience. I certainly did not always understand all of them and still can have a hard time following them (though it isn't always necessary to). It probably is necessary to assess each situation and decide what action to take. I hope the following can add to the knowledge you already have.

When you are ready, go to those people who you trust and who you think can be supportive. Friends, family, partners in love, crime, activism, etc. are the first place I thought to go. Start by telling them what you know and/or what you want them to know. You can tailor each explanation to each individual.

You may have to go beyond your initial comfort level. After my diagnosis, I struggled (and still do) with knowing who to tell and who to seek/expect support from. Aside from the first string, I also decided to tell those who I was working on projects with just so they knew the underlying reason for my change of energy and availability. Here, I also found support and understanding.

Ask for what you need. We rarely get exactly what we want, but sometimes we don't get anything even close! If you need more (or less), think of ways to ask for it. Your supporters are probably not mind readers and don't be so sure your hinting is obvious. Instead of keeping things bottled up inside, deal with the issue before it becomes larger than it has to be. Of course be reasonable with what you are asking for and from whom. But don't be shy. Have open and honest conversations about what you can do for each other to make sure you both are getting your supporter/supportee needs met. This could take the form of check-in sessions every once in a while.

Don't be afraid to say what you don't need or don't want! If you don't want to talk about your illness at the moment someone inquires, you could say something like: "it's sweet of you to ask but that topic is too draining for me right now." There will most likely be times when someone will give you unsolicited medical advice and if that annoys you, say so: "thank you for thinking of me, but I cannot take in any more information as I am consistently overwhelmed by all the choices/medicines/herbs I already have to consider."

Don't assume that you can trust someone to keep the information you share with them confidential. People tend to share information that has affected them emotionally. This is not always in a gossipy way as it could be that they are trying to help (like wanting others to know so they can support you too). Regardless of motives, it can be very frustrating. So just be clear about what information (if any) you feel comfortable with them sharing. Alternatively, it may be helpful to have people you trust explain your situation in your terms to others if you are too tired, scared, or whatever to tell them yourself. Make sure to ask if they are comfortable doing so.

Be patient. Just as we are asking for this from others, we must also give it. There are going to be people who are accustomed to giving support, but there are also going to be others who need more time or guidance. Remember, this can be a bumpy, emotional process. Just as you are getting used to a new part of your identity, so are those in your life. When in the thick of your troubles, it may seem those close to you should be feeling as emotionally connected to what's going on as you are. But in reality that is not going to be the case most of the time. This does not mean they don't think about you or want to help. Remember to ask about it if you need/want to.

Also remember that every new person who comes into your life and receives the knowledge of your illness/needs is a new place to start. While you are now familiar with your needs and the support others in your life provide, this new person is most likely not and you may need to start the process from the beginning.

Be understanding of mistakes. Beyond not being able to know what support is needed, sometimes people will do things that can come off as harsh or negligent. This could be because of the stress of your illness or other things in their life, but please don't be so quick to judge. Recognize the difficulties your supporters are encountering. Give chances and accept mistakes.

Deal constructively with their worries. My family was so worried about me early on. I understood that it was only because they cared about me, but they had to understand how it was an extra burden for me to worry about them worrying about me! So we talked it through. And while they still worry, now it's kept in check because we understand the causes and triggers for the other person. You may find that you may not even remember your self-determination when making serious, stressful decisions. But ultimately, it is your choice what you do with your body, life, mind, etc. Just be respectful and explain yourself the best you can and hope they understand.

Be patient with yourself. I am not always patient or understanding of what I perceive as my supporters' weaknesses. This may have to do with feelings of guilt for needing/expecting of them – which you should get over because you both provide things for each other. Explore these feelings to find if you should express frustration as there will be times it is most certainly justified. But before doing so, think it through and talk about it with someone else to see if you should bring it up or if it is something you might need to work on alone (first).

Assess where you are, who you're with, how much time you have and more before launching into things. I'll add a qualifier: "when you can." Of course there are going to be times you cannot hold it in and shouldn't! And those who will be there for you at all times are the best.

Give gentle reminders. Everyone forgets. Like if your friend is asking you to go on a bike ride even if you told them the other day that you can't ride a bike right now, tell them again as nicely as you can. This can be especially true with an illness that is at times invisible as it can make people (yourself included) wishfully feel as if everything is fixed and will not be bad again. This, unfortunately, may not be true. So know that after each one of these relapses you may have to start over in your illness reminders or sensitivity requests.

If their forgetting seems more like a chronic problem, rather than just an honest mistake, try to communicate about it openly. Confront them constructively with I statements like: "I feel sad when I have to remind people frequently of my new physical limitations."

There are going to be certain people with whom you may not be able to discuss your illness with or rely on support from. This is not to say they are bad friends or people and it is not that you won't still be able to have some form of a relationship with them or that this will not change. You'll probably know who these people are fairly early on. In more serious situations, you may want to decide how much you are willing to stand in case you have to make the decision to not have them in your life for certain periods or forever. Remember your right as a person and especially "as someone struggling with health issues ... to try to surround yourself with loving and nurturing people and move away from those who are just taking up your emotions" (as said by Ben, your lovely zine editor).

Be appreciative! And show it! Everyone needs reassurance they are doing the right thing. So work within your means to give your supporters the appreciation they deserve. If someone asks how you're doing and that makes you feel good, tell them! If someone bakes you gluten-free, vegan cupcakes make sure they know how much they (the person and the sweets) mean to you (thank you Tom!).

Try a support group. This may be especially useful for several reasons: you are able to talk with people who are experiencing similar things and it could act as a supplement for lack of support from friends, family, partners, etc. If there isn't one in your area that you like, start one.

Go see a counselor or therapist if you can. It's great because you can say anything you want to them! You don't have to worry about their feelings or about saying things that will affect how they react to you. Their help may not be free or easily affordable, but it might be easier than you think. Many universities have counseling services that are free if you are a student and community organizations may offer similar services to all. Search around.

Remember you. Remember who you are. You are not your illness but an amazing creature. You are changed, but you carry many of those things you always have. Remember those things when communicating with people and assessing situations.

Do something for yourself every day. It helps the spirits.

Do something for others every day. It helps the world go round.

Lastly, use what you've learned from your experience of receiving support and use it to give the best support you can to others.

That is quite a list, but certainly not exhaustive. Basically, it's about listening to each other. Being honest about our concerns and expressing gratitude. Being kind and open. As always, it's about creating a world where we all want to live. Remember: we're all in this together.

I like to think, if nothing else, these experiences with illness/death/other tough stuff help us be better supporters and supportees.

P.S. a huge thank you to Ben, Mandy and Brittany for their great feedback!

CARE FOR BODIES AND SUSTAINABLE COMMUNITIES

BETH PUMA

"So writing this is gonna be really difficult. Not difficult like riding your bike
ten miles home after you flipped over your handle bars and scraped up your
knuckles and knees but difficult like riding your bike ten miles up a hill
and knowing that taking a break from pedaling is not an option."

—Jodi Tilton, date unknown.

That is an excerpt from a poem that I didn't discover until my best friend, Jodi
Tilton, had passed away. It gives me the tiniest glimpse into her experiences living with colitis. It is because of this glimpse that I continue to think, discuss, and
read about the idea of "care."

Jodi and I became friends in 2004. She was a friend of a friend, who I had seen
around at local events and shows. I remember this mutual friend talking about
her many trips to the hospital. It wasn't until I became much closer with Jodi that
I came to realize how much colitis impacted her daily life. We became involved
with a local community organizing project called the Long Island Freespace. Our
friendship was of a care and a depth that I miss tremendously and have not been
able to recreate since her death.

For the record I do not have a chronic illness nor have I ever been diagnosed with
a serious illness. However, I am no stranger to hospitals, the disempowering at-
titudes of doctors, or daily pharmaceutical regimes. In the summer of 2007, I
watched nurse after nurse jab IV needles in my best friend's tiny veins. I had conversations with her as she began to lose motor function. I held her hand as she lay
in a hospital bed in a coma. I watched her family make the decision to terminate
life support. Perhaps I have something to say about illness-but let us rewind.

Jodi had a chronic auto immune disorder called colitis. Without going into too
much of the medical details, it affected her ability to digest food properly and
therefore absorb nutrients. When she would have flare ups, her weight would
fluctuate ten to fifteen pounds. Sometimes this required hospitalization so she

could be provided with nutrients through an IV. In January of 2007, she began to have a series of flares ups that brought her to the decision to take a prescribed steroid, something she had always avoided. Because of the intense mood swings and other side effects of these drugs, she was prescribed various anti-anxiety and sleep aids. Fed up with the amount of pills that her doctors were pushing, she eventually chose to take an experimental medication in June that was an intravenous treatment. Her family and friends do not know the exact connection between this and what happened, but within a month she was hospitalized and within two weeks of that she passed away.

I think about the mistakes I made. I ask myself 'was I a good enough friend? Were there things I could have done differently?' My personal answers to those questions are just that —personal—but her death has gotten me thinking about communities and support.

A common cry we have in radical communities is "be the change you want to see" or "a new world is possible." What does this look like? I am tired of the same sorry blanket response of "whatever you want it to be." I am in search of a very practical, compassionate and effective approach to dealing with illness (and other areas where support is needed, such as death, acts of violence, etc.) People within my community are getting older, some of them have been diagnosed with conditions that affect their day to day living. Some have battled cancer or other serious diseases.

The first thing I learned from Jodi is in order to be a supportive friend it is imperative not to ignore a friend's illness. There were times when Jodi's illness was like an elephant that many people chose to ignore. A group of us would be out for drinks or at dinner, and she was not able to eat or drink while others enjoyed in the gluttony. Sometimes there was no acknowledgement that she had not been eating because her illness would not allow her to hold her food down or would cause painful diarrhea. She hated that. In addition there were even friends who in not knowing what to say, said nothing at all-and eventually grew distant and allowed the friendship to fizzle. Jodi was incredibly loyal to her friends and it made her illness so much more painful (quite literally because it was compounded by stress) to have experiences like walking by someone on the street who used to be a close friend without any acknowledgement.

Another thing that I learned from Jodi is to understand the difference between being a good listener, and keeping your two cents to yourself. Asking the question "how are you feeling?" without real sincerity is half-assed and frustrating. Jodi used to hate that question. "I feel like shit ok ... do you want to hear about it?" was the response she always wished she could say. Being a good listener isn't easy, depending on the severity of the illness, it can be exhausting. I watched my friend Jodi struggle for six months before deciding to go on the new treatment. I would listen to her as she expressed frustration because of people she considered friends who did not return *phone call after phone call*. In addition, it is not really helpful to offer up advice to an illness that one doesn't know anything about. Telling a person with colitis to drink ginger ale to help their stomach problems is frustrating at best and patronizing at worst. If Jodi wanted my voice, she asked for it. By being a good listener, you don't impose on the person with illness's voice.

In addition, I believe if we are trying to create systems outside of capitalism and other systems of oppression, supporting friends with illnesses has to be more organized. The weight and task of supporting friends cannot fall solely onto the shoulders of a partner and/or best friend. We have to take these discussions outside the realm of whispers and late night phone calls of suffering. Besides being isolating for the person fighting illness, it leads to burnout of the closest in contact-and therefore is not sustainable. We should also ask ourselves, 'Is the act of CARE falling to the gender most often associated with care?' That is also not sustainable in addition to falling into the systems of oppression that many of us work against. It is the role of the community (and the test of one) to walk beside those of us who are fighting.

Though undoubtedly incomplete, the following are a few additional ideas on community effort that needs to take place when one of our own falls ill.

In the case of hospitalization, groups of people can gather goods in the form of a gift basket. Hospitals are weird places. Having a toothbrush, some soap, and deodorant (and a book) makes the experience a little easier. This should not be the sole responsibility of any person. This is the easiest of collective endeavors.

Based on the needs of the person in the hospital, is someone visiting at least once a day? The person hospitalized may not want visitors all the time, or they may. If it is the case where they enjoy the company of friends (sometimes it is a welcome distraction to the doting of parents) then people should coordinate with their work schedules to swing by, if even for twenty minutes. I recommend bringing a favorite food or slice of cake, if medically possible, because hospital food is gross, especially if the person is vegetarian or vegan.

Let's say a person isn't hospitalized but is home bound after a treatment or flare up. Sometimes day to day routine becomes super exhausting. Cooking a meal for a friend is a way of keeping them company and meeting their nutritional needs. Depending on the needs and desires of the person working through their illness this should be organized in a way to share the labor. One person takes Monday, another can take Wednesday, another Friday, etc — or whatever meets the needs of the person. Maybe the person's dietary needs are taken care of, but is their laundry, errands, or even grocery shopping handled?

Let me stop and say that I feel these are simple ideas. Share the labor. Duh. People should take turns providing care. Duh. These are elementary ideas, but I wish I would see them more. I think about ways that we could have better served my friend Jodi in her illness. But what really got me thinking again even more ardently about this idea of community care is how the same fucking mistakes were being repeated as other friends battled sickness. **So if what I'm saying seems elementary, then I ask my community and myself, 'Why are we not doing it?'**

Another way that we can support our friends as a community is by holding people accountable. Some may say this is a "call out" process. I would prefer to say it is a way to challenge those we surround ourselves with. I can't count the amount of times that Jodi would be expressing her frustrations to me on the phone about feeling rejected or ignored by her friends simply because of her illness. It is hard to find the words for a friend who is ill but habitually refusing to say anything is **just unacceptable.** More than her body failing her, this is what hurt Jodi the most-**being ignored.** This is where as a community we can be better. We need to reach out to each other through our own methods of self organization and remind people how their actions are hurtful. **We need to reach out to each other to push ourselves through uncomfortableness in order to best support a friend.**

Finally, continuing these discussions as they are applicable to our respective communities is super helpful. Providing people who fight disease and illness the avenue to share/vent/kick/scream/ educate is a valuable tool.

I am aging. My friends are getting older. Our bodies are changing and there will be more of us who will come across health complications that come with age. The fact still remains that there are some of us within our communities who have been dealing with health conditions for a long time. These questions are not going to go away. I came up with some thoughts and plans of action and I am sure that there are many ideas out there. More than anything I just offer the challenge to be more conscious of community activity in terms of how we care for our members.

TIPS FOR BEING A "PATIENT"

BEN HOLTZMAN

Dealing with a serious medical condition can be overwhelming. In trying to manage your health and wellness, you have to process information that comes at you from various directions and make major decisions about your health and care. Few of us have even thought about ever being in this position and fewer still have models for how to do so.

In the following, I have noted some things I found particularly helpful in being a "patient" (i.e. the aspect of illness that involves dealing with doctors). In my case, I've mostly dealt with cancer doctors, but I've also tried to incorporate perspectives from people who are dealing with other serious health conditions. This is by no means exhaustive or applicable to all situations, so please take the suggestions that are helpful and disregard the rest.

One of the most important parts of being a patient is remembering to be understanding and kind to yourself. Dealing with a serious health condition is difficult in so many ways. There are plenty of good things that come out of dealing with doctors, but also lots of things that can be, well, less than pleasant. Remember that you are not the first person to feel frustrated by the process. Be patient with yourself and give yourself credit for every step you take!

If you're newly diagnosed, you will probably need to find a doctor who is going to treat you (who in many cases may be different from the one who diagnosed you). The extent to which you have a choice about this can be limited by resources, insurance, finances, and time, but if you have the means, try to find the person in whose hands you are going to feel the most comfortable. Some people find it helpful to approach this as if they are "hiring" a doctor who is the best person for the job (this might be a difficult analogy for radicals with an aversion to being a boss!) This could mean the person who is known as the "expert" in the field or the person who was recommended by someone you trust or some combination of factors, but the important thing is to try to find the person who you are most comfortable receiving care from.

This may involve seeking out a second or even third opinion. Again, the extent to which you can do this may be limited. Even if you have insurance and it allows for this, it is not always easy: finding a second opinion can involve jumping through hoops to figure out who to see, clearing each step with your insurance, accessing your medical records, making sure the new doctor/hospital has all the information that they need for the appointment, and potentially travelling out of your area for the appointment. But another opinion can change the trajectory of your care and put you in hands you feel more comfortable with.

Dealing with an illness typically means having a lot of doctor appointments. It can be really useful to keep a single notepad to write down all of the important information that you receive as well as a single binder or folder to keep track of all of your important documents. This way, all of your relevant information can stay in one place.

A notebook is particularly helpful in doctor's appointments. In high stress situations where you are dealing with lots of new information, your ability to process information and remember it can be hindered, so writing down important information can be critical.

It can also be really useful to go over your notes after an appointment. I have sometimes found that I thought I understood what a doctor told me during an appointment but in going over my notes or explaining what was said to someone else, I realized that I had questions that did not hit me during the appointment.

I also found it really useful to keep a running list of questions that would come up in between appointments. Of course, there were some questions that could not wait and for those I had to call the doctor. But for a lot of others, I could wait until the next appointment and wouldn't always remember them unless I wrote them down.

I strongly recommend bringing someone into appointments with you. Ideally, this would be the same person each time so that you have at least one person who is always keeping track of the same information that you are. When I was first diagnosed, my parents (who were separated but both lived nearby) insisted on coming with me to my appointments. I was REALLY resistant to this idea. I think that going on my own made me feel like I had control over what was happening and that the situation was something I could handle. In retrospect, I am extremely thankful that I got over this. I found that, particularly in the beginning, when the doctor went over results and recommendations, it felt like watching a movie in fast forward. I tried to understand and catch what I could, but the information inevitably came out in a way that became hard for me to always process, never mind catch the minutia of. Having at least one other person in the room to hear this information and to ask questions was extremely useful. It also became really important for us to talk after the appointment. I was amazed how often one of us had understood something the doctor said slightly differently than the other. Being able to clarify points and come up with additional questions was very useful in ensuring that I fully understood what was happening with my health and treatment.

If you do not have someone to come with you, you may want to bring a tape recorder into appointments with you. This way, you have a record of what the doctor said and can easily clarify any questions.

As we all know, doctors can be difficult to deal with. Experiences can vary vastly with different doctors, but quite often, patients are kept waiting past appointment times, doctors can speak at a level that is difficult to understand, patients can be made to feel like they are taking up the doctor's precious time if they ask questions, etc. Do not be afraid to ask doctors all the questions that you have before leaving your appointment or to ask them to rephrase things so that you are sure you know what they are saying. Also, try not to be shy about your feelings and apprehensions when talking with your doctor; your doctor should know what you're thinking.

When discussing treatment options, do not be afraid to ask what options might be possible other than the one the doctor is recommending (if this is information you want to know). Also, if you are unsure about what option to pursue, see if it would be possible to call the doctor the next day to make a decision (if time allows), rather than being pressured into the decision during the appointment.

You may find it helpful to do research about your condition on your own. I would have thought that doctors and hospitals would have provided me with significant information about my condition and what was going to happen, along with recommendations for reading more on my own, but it was actually the opposite. They really only told me what they felt I needed to know (which was generally a bare minimum). But doing research on your own can be tricky. After being diagnosed, one of the first things I came across in trying to do research was a list of people who had died from the type of cancer that I had. I decided right then to hold off on any additional research. Over time, it became easier to read more about my condition, but especially in the beginning, I really relied mostly on what doctors said. Of course, it is important to be well informed, but there may be limits to the information you want to expose yourself to. If you find it difficult to do research on your own but are interested in learning more than what the doctor is telling you, you may want to ask someone you trust to do research for you. This person can filter out the misleading, frightening, and bizarre stuff you can come across and only pass along the information that is useful.

One last word about dealing with doctors: some people feel the need to research all aspects of their conditions and are never afraid to question doctors about what they find. Others do not have any desire to learn more than what their doctor is telling them and need to put their faith in their doctor's hands in order to get through their situation. Neither approach is better than the other. You can only do what you feel you are capable of and however you choose to handle your illness and treatment in order to get yourself through it is the right way.

Of course, there are lots of other aspects of getting through these experiences that do not involve doctors. I am just going to touch on a few suggestions below:

Consider keeping a journal. This can give you a space to express yourself in a way that you may not be able to (or may not want to) with others. It can be really cathartic in dealing with all of the mess involved in having an illness. You may also find it useful to try certain exercises during tougher times like the one mentioned in the zine, *Support*: "write down everything you can think of that is beautiful, that makes you feel alive, or that you simply *like*."

Consider seeing a therapist. Most people don't talk enough about the emotional side of dealing with illness, but this can be just as hard, if not harder, than the physical. Therapy can be really helpful.

One last suggestion: don't be afraid of indulgence. If you're battling a serious health condition, don't be afraid to treat yourself every once in a while (or more than that!). You deserve it. Indulgence can take many forms from buying yourself a record you've always wanted to finally ridding yourself of the negative, energy-sucking vampires in your life. Maybe even consider making a list of all of the things that you want to do and still can do and do them!

Though dealing with illness will always be tough, it is possible to maintain a semblance of control and even to feel empowered in navigating through the world of doctors and medicine. Remember to recognize all of the steps you take in living your life while dealing with illness. Appreciate your own efforts, give yourself kudos, and love yourself for being so brave.

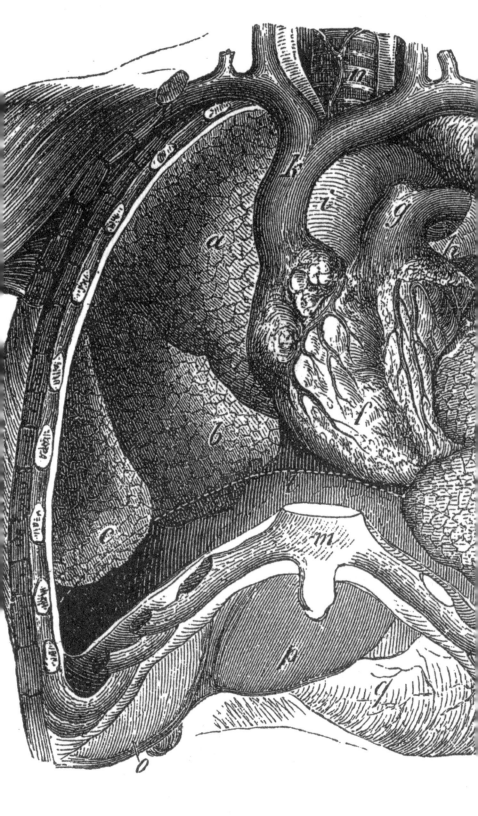

BIOS:

Emiko Badillo was born in 1975 to a Mexican dad and a Japanese mom. Being sick is the cherry on top of the crazy sundae that is her life. With the support of great friends, parents, brothers, and her husband, Chad, and dog, Ago, she continues to live and have fun.

Joe Biel is a videomaker, author, zinester, tea drinker, publisher, bicycle mechanic, electrician, organizer, patch sewer, and recently converted cell phone user. He is currently working on a book of interviews for Garrett County Press with old punks who pursued things other than music. He doesn't know where he lives.

Krista Ciminera lives and works in Brooklyn, NY. Half of her time is spent riding her bike, and the other half is spent as a feminist activist in the For The Birds Collective, playing guitar in Zombie Dogs, and learning as much as she can.

Lauren Denitzio is an illustrator and graphic designer living in Brooklyn, currently self-employed and playing in the band The Measure [sa]. She grew up in New Jersey and was diagnosed with Marfan Syndrome, a connective tissue disorder, as a young child. She is a member of the For The Birds feminist collective and distro and enjoys writing music and drawing. She is interested in talking to more people about similar illnesses and can be reached at lauren.denitzio@gmail.com.

Mandy Earley is an editorial associate working in academic publishing in Durham, NC. She loves reading and writing about radical politics, consumer culture, medicine, and health care. More of her writing can be found on her blog LOVE/SICKNESS: http://radicalrx.blogspot.com. Feel free to write Mandy at jennylain@gmail.com if you'd like to discuss the topics presented here, on the blog, or any other aspects of sick life.

ema has a strong midwestern heart and a love of tiny things and insects. Appreciation often overwhelms her, in a good way. She dislikes illness but likes what we can learn from it. She wishes for a world where people always are good to each other and where there are no prisons.

Erica lives in Durham, NC and goes to UNC Chapel Hill for social work. She was diagnosed with Crohn's colitis (an autoimmune disease of the colon) when she was 16. Aside from paying medical bills and fighting with insurance companies, Erica likes to sing, play her trombone and kazoo, and be crafty with paper and fabric. Her favorite color is green.

Ben Holtzman's work has appeared in *Clamor Magazine*, *Journal of Popular Music Studies*, *Left History*, *Maximumrocknroll*, *Popular Music and Society*, *Radical Society* and the collections *Constituent Imagination* (AK Press) and *In The Middle of a Whirlwind* (JOAAP). He has wanted to do a zine since *Maximumrocknroll* first made his fingers black at age twelve, but never would have guessed it'd be on this topic. Be in touch with him through: illnesszine@gmail.com

Sarah Hughes is a New York City Public School teacher and ABA Therapist, originally from Austin, Texas. Hughes is a proud member of the Park Slope Food Cooperative, Teachers Unite and is an avid crafter. This is Hughes's first zine contribution, and she can be reached at: sarah.scatterheart@gmail.com

Emily Klamer is a student, writer, and activist from Missouri. Her passions include advocating for survivors of sexual and intimate partner violence, cultivating a feminist praxis, and remembering how to have fun. Notes can be sent to emmylou@riseup.net

Luci lives in Columbia, MO. She spends her free time doing bizarre things like studying toxicology, collecting comic books, and spending 3 hours daily playing pool so she can eventually hustle suckers. After her heart transplant, she plans to move to Olympia, WA to become a mountain climbing guide. Please feel free to contact her through: theonlythingtofearis_fear@yahoo.com

Kristin Alysia Pape has been swallowed whole by an endless PhD dissertation about the "ailing body" in film and literature, but escapes routinely enough to teach writing and visual/cultural studies at Pratt Institute. She lives (and obsessively knits) in Brooklyn with her partner and a menagerie of variously-disabled animals.

Tessa Petrocco is an Ohio-born freelance writer currently based out of New York City. Her work can be seen on Spill.com as well as Shockya.com. She has been embracing her "pimp walk" since 1993 and is secretly happy she has a valid excuse to own a handicapped parking decal.

Beth Puma is a former resident of Brooklyn, NY who has relocated to sunny Tucson. She is a public school teacher. She was involved with the Long Island Freespace and the Long Island Womyn's Collective. There she organized with Jodi Tilton, the friend she writes about here and whom she still grieves over. Currently, Beth is pursuing various writing adventures. She is also a guinea pig enthusiast and loves to talk to folks about that as well.

Rachel is a double aquarius who enjoys most things with wings, vegan cooking/eating, and pumping iron. When not tackling the demands of graduate school she can most often be found snuggling with her cats, smooshy and liam, and watching 90210 reruns.

Rainbow was diagnosed with chronic kidney disease when she was 2 years old. She received a kidney from her mother in 2001, and is now focusing on staying healthy, being creative, going to college, and making a life for herself.

Andrea Runyan is a recent Stanford graduate in math and biology. She is currently working from home as Lyme disease project manager. In her free time, she makes use of the Cambridge public library network and writes on HubPages and her Lyme blog (freeideasblog.blogspot.com). She aims to be a health and spirituality writer. She thanks her Dad, Mom and boyfriend for their support. She can be reached at monandreamichelle@gmail.com

Brittany Shoot is an American writer and activist based in Copenhagen, Denmark. She and her partner live with their cat Malcolm and attempt to be vegan in an omnivorous country. Acupuncture and herbal therapy have drastically reduced the frequency of and pain associated with her migraines. She is working on her first solo zine about life in Denmark.

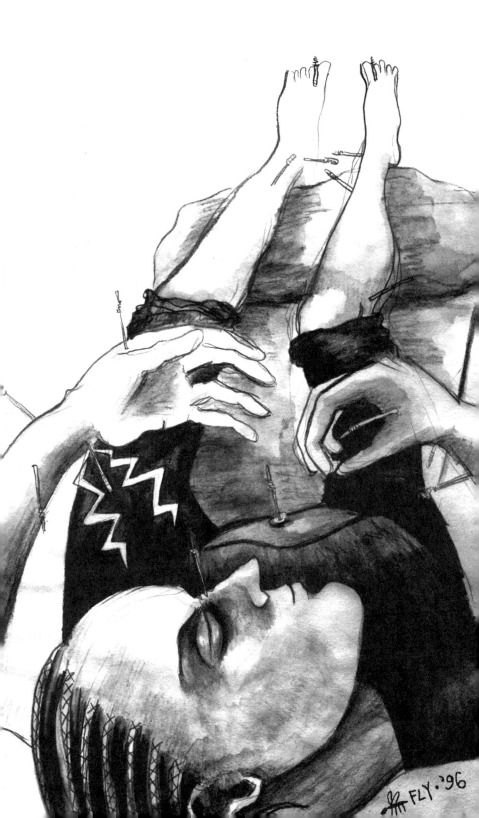

FLY.'96

RESOURCE LIST:

SUPPORT AND CAREGIVING

The Etiquette of Illness: What To Say When You Can't Find The Words (Susan P. Halpern)

Help Me Live: 20 Things People With Cancer Want You To Know (Lori Hope)

An Uncertain Inheritance: Writers on Caring for Family (Nell Casey)

"The Importance of Support: Building Foundations, Sustaining Community," Rolling Thunder: An Anarchist Journal of Dangerous Living Issue 6 (Fall 2008), 29-39. Soon to be revised, expanded and published as a pamphlet by PM Press

ILLNESS/DISABILITY

The Cancer Journals (Audrey Lorde)

The Natural Remedy Book for Women (Diane Stein)

The Patient's Voice: Experiences Of Illness (Jeanine Young-Mason)

Waist-High in the World: A Life Among the Nondisabled (Nancy Mairs)

"All of Our Lives: Renewing the Social Model of Disability" (Liz Crow)

http://www.roaring-girl.com/socialmodel.pdf

ZINES (THESE ALL TOUCH ON ILLNESS AND RELATED ISSUES)

About My Disappearance (#1-2)

Broken Hipster (#1-3)

Caboose (#6)

Harlot, RN

May Cause Dizziness

Suzie is a Robot

When Language Runs Dry: A Zine for People with Chronic Pain and Their Allies

WEBSITES ON ILLNESS/DISABILITY

www.healingwell.com - HealingWell Forum

www.mdjunction.com - MD Junction: Online Support Groups for Your Health Challenges

PERSONAL SUSTAINABILITY AND HEALTH

Aftershock: Confronting Trauma in a Violent World - A Guide for Activists and Their Allies (Pattrice Jones)

Counterbalance: Thoughts on Activism and Mental Health

FOOD/DIET

The Allergy Self-Help Cookbook (Marjorie Hurt Jones)

What to Eat When You Can't Eat Anything (Chupi Sweetman)

DEATH AND GRIEF

Loss: The Politics of Mourning (David L. Eng and David Kazanjian)

The Worst: A Compilation Zine on Grief and Loss

MENTAL HEALTH

Bay Area Radical Mental Health Collective (www.radicalmentalhealth.net)

The Icarus Project (theicarusproject.net)

BE OUR "BEST FRIEND FOREVER

Just like supporting your local farmers, we now offer a "subscription" to everything that we publish! Every time we publish something new we'll send it to your door! Perfect for people who love to get a monthly package but don't have time to sift through what they want!

Minimum subscription period is 6 months. Subscription begins the month after it is purchased. To receive more than 6 months, add multiple orders to your quantity.

Sliding Scale $15-30/month, based on what you can afford!

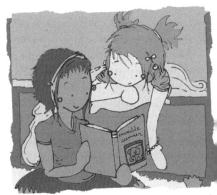

www.microcosmpublishing.com/
catalog/other/2241/0

Microcosm Publishing
222 S Rogers St. Bloomington, IN 47404
www.microcosmpublishing.com